Good Bones Healthy Bones

Natural Remedies to Treat Osteoporosis

Forward

To all who suffer from osteoporosis this is the reason I wrote this book. I wrote this book after being diagnosed with osteoporosis. After researching the negative effects of traditional medications, I decided did not want the side effects from such medications, so I am writing this book to inform you of safer and alternative natural solutions.

I am beginning my journey on this quest for good bone density. But for what I have been doing I wanted to share with you the safe results of dealing with this naturally. I am fortunate to have a doctor who is working with me on my quest for natural solutions to osteoporosis. My advice is to work with a doctor of Osteopathy (D.O.). They are more open to natural methods in medicine.

Buy organic I can't encourage you enough because farmers these days use completely too many pesticides with no regard to our health. You can't

wash all the pesticides off and we eat poison if we
don't buy organic.

Marcia
Durbin

Chapter 1 Understanding Osteoporosis

Bones provide the framework for our bodies, a crucial foundation that supports movement and protects vital organs. Yet, for millions of people worldwide, this framework can become dangerously fragile due to osteoporosis. Imagine a scenario where a simple fall or even a minor bump results in a broken hip or wrist. This isn't just a distant possibility for those with osteoporosis; it's an ever-present risk. The quiet progression of this bone disease often goes unnoticed until a sudden fracture changes everything, highlighting the importance of understanding its causes and impact on bone health.

Osteoporosis is more than just a condition of weakened bones; it's a complex interplay of various factors that compromise skeletal strength. Genetics, for instance, play a significant role, determining one's predisposition to lower bone mass and density. Such inherited vulnerabilities are beyond one's control but acknowledging them can prompt timely interventions and preventive measures. Lifestyle choices add another layer of complexity. Habits like smoking and excessive alcohol consumption negatively influence bone health, reducing calcium absorption and disrupting hormonal balances essential for maintaining strong bones. Add to this the risks associated with a sedentary lifestyle, certain medical conditions, and medications that weaken bones, and it becomes evident that osteoporosis is a multifaceted issue requiring comprehensive management.

In this chapter, we will delve into the numerous factors contributing to osteoporosis and their interrelations. From genetic predispositions to lifestyle decisions, we'll explore how each element plays a part in bone health deterioration. Furthermore, we will discuss preventive strategies, including dietary adjustments, physical activities, and necessary lifestyle modifications, to help mitigate these risks.

Consulting healthcare providers and undergoing regular screenings will also be emphasized as critical steps for early detection and effective management of osteoporosis. By understanding these dimensions, readers will be equipped with the knowledge needed to adopt proactive measures for maintaining robust bone health.

Factors Contributing to Osteoporosis

Understanding osteoporosis starts with recognizing what this bone disease entails and its profound impact on bone health. Osteoporosis occurs when bones become weak and brittle, to the extent that a minor bump or a simple fall can lead to fractures, most commonly in the hip, wrist, and spine (Branch, 2017). It's often called a "silent" disease because it progresses without symptoms until a fracture happens.

Genetics and family history play a significant role in predisposing individuals to osteoporosis. Your genetic makeup can influence your bone mass and density, which are critical factors in bone strength. If you have a family history of osteoporosis or fractures, particularly hip fractures
among your parents, you may be at a higher risk yourself (Mayo Clinic, 2024). While understanding your genetic predisposition is important for awareness and early detection, it is an area we can't control directly. But acknowledging this risk can push us toward more frequent screenings and preventive measures.

Lifestyle choices also significantly impact bone health. Smoking and excessive alcohol consumption have both been shown to negatively affect bone density. Smoking interferes with the body's ability to use calcium efficiently, leading to lower bone mass. Similarly, excessive alcohol consumption can disrupt the balance of calcium by affecting the hormones related to bone health and decreasing the absorption of nutrients essential for bone integrity (Pouresmaeili et al., 2018).

Here is what you can do to mitigate these risks:

- Quit smoking if you currently smoke, or avoid starting if you don't.

- Limit alcohol consumption to moderate levels. For women, this means no more than one drink per day; for men, no more than two drinks per day.

- Engage in weight-bearing physical activities such as walking, jogging, or dancing, which help strengthen bones.

A sedentary lifestyle exacerbates the risk of developing osteoporosis. Bones need regular exercise to stay healthy and robust. Engaging in regular physical activity stimulates the formation of new bone tissue and helps maintain bone density. Conversely, lack of physical activity leads to bone loss and higher susceptibility to fractures (Branch, 2017).

Another factor not to overlook is the impact of certain medical conditions and medications on bone health. Conditions such as rheumatoid arthritis, celiac disease, and hormonal imbalances can weaken bones over time. Long-term use of corticosteroids and other medications used to treat chronic diseases can interfere with the bone-rebuilding process, increasing the risk of osteoporosis (Goh et al., 2018).

Consulting with healthcare providers about potential risk factors is crucial for prevention. They can guide you on:

- The necessity of bone density tests if you have a condition or medication that might weaken your bones.

- Alternative treatments that might have less impact on bone health.

- Supplementation and lifestyle changes tailored to counteract the bone-weakening effects of your condition or medications.

Nutritional factors hold substantial importance in maintaining strong bones. Calcium and vitamin D are particularly critical. Calcium is the building block of bone tissue, while vitamin D enhances calcium absorption in the gut. A diet low in these nutrients can compromise bone strength and increase the risk of osteoporosis. Consuming adequate amounts of these nutrients throughout life can help preserve bone density and reduce the likelihood of fractures (Mayo Clinic, 2024).

To ensure you're getting enough calcium and vitamin D:

- Incorporate calcium-rich foods into your diet, including dairy products, green leafy vegetables, canned salmon, and fortified cereals. • Spend some time outdoors each day to help your body produce vitamin D from sunlight. If you live in a high latitude, are housebound, or regularly use sunscreen, consider vitamin D supplements.

- Opt for foods fortified with vitamin D, such as milk and cereals, to support your dietary intake.

Beyond these individual factors, it's beneficial to adopt a holistic approach to bone health. For those living with osteoporosis or seeking to prevent it, integrating multiple strategies can offer the best protection. Combining a nutrient-rich diet, regular physical activity, and lifestyle modifications like quitting smoking and limiting alcohol can collectively fortify bone health and mitigate risks.

Regular screenings for bone density, especially if you fall into high-risk categories—such as having a family history of osteoporosis or being postmenopausal—are essential. Early detection through bone density tests can identify osteoporosis before a fracture occurs, allowing for timely intervention.

In summary, while osteoporosis stems from various controllable and uncontrollable factors, taking proactive steps can significantly reduce the risk of developing the disease or mitigating its impact. Understanding your genetic predisposition, making positive lifestyle changes, consulting healthcare providers about potential risks, and ensuring nutritional adequacy in calcium and vitamin D are all integral strategies in maintaining strong bone health.

It's evident that personal responsibility combined with a supportive safety net is vital in addressing osteoporosis effectively. By leveraging empirical evidence and data-driven insights, we can better navigate the complexities of this silent disease, prioritizing human welfare alongside economic considerations. This balanced approach ensures that our actions today lead to healthier bones and improved quality of life in the future.

The Importance of Bone Density

Bone density is a critical indicator of skeletal health, influencing fracture risk and overall mobility. Essentially, bone density reflects the amount of minerals, primarily calcium and phosphate, within your bones, contributing to their strength and rigidity. When bone density decreases, bones become porous and fragile, akin to a honeycomb structure, which significantly heightens the susceptibility to fractures.

Age-related bone density loss is a natural process, particularly post-menopause for women, but certain lifestyle choices can accelerate this decline. Importantly, engaging in bone-strengthening activities can help maintain optimal bone density. Here are a few strategies to consider:

- Integrate weight-bearing exercises, such as walking, jogging, and climbing stairs into your routine. These activities force your bones to work against gravity, stimulating bone growth.

- Incorporate resistance training, like lifting weights or using resistance bands, to enhance muscle strength and pressure on bones.

- Ensure adequate intake of bone-friendly nutrients, especially calcium and vitamin D, to support bone health.

- Avoid smoking and limit alcohol consumption as these habits can weaken bone structure.

- Consider medication if prescribed by a healthcare professional to aid in maintaining bone density.

Low bone density is often asymptomatic until fractures occur, underscoring the importance of preventive measures. Early detection through screening tests is essential for timely intervention. Osteoporosis, for instance, typically remains silent until it manifests through fractures, often when a simple fall creates a break that would not have ordinarily caused significant harm.

For early detection, it's vital to undergo regular screening tests, such as DEXA scans. These dual-energy X-ray absorptiometry scans are non-invasive and measure bone mineral density (BMD). The test compares your bone density with the expected BMD for healthy young adults and helps evaluate your risk of fractures. By identifying low bone density early, you can take proactive steps to prevent severe damage.

The relevance of DEXA scans cannot be overstated. This tool provides a comprehensive picture of your bone health status, highlighting areas that require attention. Regular monitoring via DEXA scans can track changes in bone density over time, enabling you and your healthcare provider to adjust your treatment plan as needed. Specifically, the results from these scans can guide decisions regarding dietary adjustments, exercise routines, and possible medical interventions like medications designed to strengthen bones.

Beyond exercise and screenings, ensuring a diet rich in calcium and vitamin D is crucial. Calcium supports bone hardness, while vitamin D enhances calcium absorption. Foods like dairy products, leafy greens, and fortified cereals are excellent calcium sources. For vitamin D, exposure to sunlight and consuming fatty fish or fortified milk can be beneficial.

Physical activity remains an appealing alternative to medication due to its reduced cost, fewer side effects, and added health benefits, including improved balance and reduced falls (Carter et al., 2014). Additionally, activities such as tennis, basketball, or even brisk walking can engender significant improvements in bone density by subjecting the skeletal frame to stress, which prompts bone formation and fortification (Carter et al., 2014).

Moreover, regular physical activities can notably increase bone size, cortical area, and strength, reducing hip fracture risks later in life. Activities should be weight-bearing and endured regularly—three to five times a week—and complemented with resistance exercises two to three times a week (Carter et al., 2014).

It's important to remember that maintaining bone health is a lifelong commitment. After peak bone mass is reached around age 30, the focus should shift towards slowing the rate of bone loss and maintaining bone strength through consistent lifestyle choices. As emphasized, a balanced diet, regular exercise, avoiding detrimental habits, and undergoing periodic bone density tests form the backbone of a robust strategy to prevent osteoporosis and related complications.

The practical implications are clear; integrating these guidelines into daily routines can lead to substantial long-term benefits. Given the often asymptomatic nature of osteoporosis, being proactive is key.

In summary, understanding the role of bone density in overall skeletal health is paramount. With age-related declines inevitable, a proactive approach involving regular exercise, a nutrient-rich diet, lifestyle adjustments, and routine DEXA scans can make a significant difference. These collective efforts ensure that bone health is maintained, preventing fractures and promoting mobility for years to come.

Steps Toward Better Bone Health

Understanding osteoporosis and its profound impact on bone health has been the central theme of this chapter. We began by recognizing osteoporosis as a "silent" disease that weakens bones to the point where minor incidents can cause severe fractures. With age, especially post-menopause for women, the risk becomes more pronounced due to the natural decline in bone density.

A return to our earlier discussion highlights that genetics and family history are uncontrollable factors contributing significantly to one's predisposition to osteoporosis. However, acknowledging these risks can lead to proactive measures such as more frequent screenings and preventive habits aimed at mitigating their effects.

Medical conditions and medications present another layer of complexity in the management of bone health. Conditions like rheumatoid arthritis and long-term use of corticosteroids can jeopardize bone strength. Consulting healthcare providers about the potential impacts of these conditions and medications is crucial. Such consultations can guide you toward alternatives or additional treatments that lessen the adverse effects on your bones.

Dietary considerations, specifically the intake of calcium and vitamin D, cannot be overlooked. These nutrients are foundational to building and maintaining strong bones. Ensuring an adequate supply of these through diet or supplements helps support bone density and overall bone health, especially as natural absorption mechanisms wane with age.

Readers should be concerned about the practical implications of these insights. Osteoporosis often remains undetected until a fracture occurs, underscoring the need for early detection through regular bone density screenings such as DEXA scans. These tests provide invaluable data that can inform personalized prevention and treatment strategies.

On a wider scale, the understanding and proactive management of osteoporosis extend beyond individual well-being to societal impact. Healthier bones mean fewer fractures, which translates to reduced healthcare costs and improved quality of life for aging populations. Therefore, it is crucial to integrate multiple strategies—diet, exercise, medical consultations, and lifestyle modifications—to create a comprehensive approach to bone health.

Ending with a thought to ponder: while we may not have control over every aspect affecting our bone health, leveraging knowledge and making informed choices today can pave the way for stronger bones and a healthier future. This holistic approach empowers individuals to take charge of their bone health, ensuring mobility and vitality in the years to come.

References

Pouresmaeili, F., Kamalidehghan, B., Kamarehei, M., Goh, Y. M. (2018). *A comprehensive overview on osteoporosis and its risk factors. Therapeutics and Clinical Risk Management*, 14, 2029. https://doi.org/10.2147/TCRM.S138000

Carter, M. I., & Hinton, P. S. (2014). *Physical activity and bone health. Missouri Medicine*, 111(1), 59. https://www.ncbi.nlm.nih.gov/pmc/articles/PMC6179512/

Mayo Clinic. (2024). *Osteoporosis - Symptoms and causes. Mayo Clinic*. Retrieved from https://www.mayoclinic.org/diseases-conditions/osteoporosis/symptoms-causes/syc-20351968

National Institute of Arthritis and Musculoskeletal and Skin Diseases. (2017). *Osteoporosis*.
Retrieved from https://www.niams.nih.gov/health-topics/osteoporosis

Mayo Clinic Staff. (2022). *Bone density test. Mayo Clinic*. Retrieved from https://www.mayoclinic.org/tests-procedures/bone-density-test/about/pac-20385273

Office of the Surgeon General (US). (2004). *Determinants of Bone Health. Bone Health and Osteoporosis*. Retrieved from https://www.ncbi.nlm.nih.gov/books/NBK45503/

Chapter 2

Natural Remedies for Osteoporosis

When it comes to managing osteoporosis, many individuals are seeking effective alternatives to conventional medications. Natural remedies are increasingly finding their place in the spotlight, offering hope to those looking for holistic approaches to improve bone health. These remedies, including herbal supplements and lifestyle changes, promise a natural alignment with the body's needs while minimizing side effects. Exploring these avenues can open up new possibilities for enhancing bone density and overall well-being.

Osteoporosis is a condition characterized by weak and brittle bones, making them susceptible to fractures even with minor falls or bumps. This ailment predominantly affects older adults, particularly postmenopausal women, due to hormonal changes that exacerbate bone loss. Traditional treatments often involve medications that may not suit everyone, owing to potential side effects and individual health considerations. Taking a more natural route with remedies like herbal supplements offers an alternative that aligns more closely with the body's inherent healing processes. For instance, herbs like turmeric and Boswellia are known for their anti-inflammatory properties, which can help reduce inflammation and support bone strength without the adverse effects associated with some pharmaceuticals.

In this chapter, we delve into a variety of natural remedies that can aid in treating osteoporosis and improving bone density. We will explore the benefits of various herbal supplements, such as turmeric, Boswellia, ginseng, and ashwagandha, highlighting how they contribute to bone health. Additionally, we will examine the roles of minerals found in herbs like horsetail and nettle, which are crucial for maintaining bone density. The chapter also covers the importance of integrating these supplements into a broader lifestyle strategy, emphasizing diet, exercise, and regular medical consultation. By understanding and applying these natural remedies, individuals can take proactive steps towards better bone health and enhanced quality of life.

Herbal Supplements for Bone Health

Herbal supplements can play a significant role in the treatment of osteoporosis. Owing to their natural composition and minimal side effects, they offer an alternative that aligns well with both individualized care and evidence-based practices. By considering personal health concerns and utilizing effective herbal remedies, we can strike a balance between economic growth and human welfare.

Turmeric and Boswellia: Anti-inflammatory Powerhouses

Turmeric and Boswellia are renowned for their potent anti-inflammatory properties. These herbs are particularly beneficial in reducing inflammation within bones, thereby promoting healing and enhancing bone strength. Turmeric, with its active compound curcumin, has demonstrated significant ability to reduce inflammatory markers. Boswellia, on the other hand, contains Boswellia acids, which have been shown to inhibit pro-inflammatory enzymes.

Here's what you can do to integrate these into your regimen:

- Consult with a healthcare provider to determine appropriate dosages.

- Incorporate turmeric powder into meals or take curcumin supplements.

- Use Boswellia extract according to recommended guidelines by a specialist.

Adaptogenic Herbs: Ginseng and Ashwagandha

Adaptogens like ginseng and ashwagandha help the body cope with stress, which can be a contributing factor in osteoporosis. Chronic stress releases cortisol, a hormone that can lead to bone density reduction over time. Ginseng enhances overall vitality and supports bodily functions, making it a valuable ally in combating osteoporosis. Similarly, ashwagandha is known to improve bone mineral density and reduce stress-related hormonal imbalances.

These steps can help you to utilize these adaptogens effectively:

- Seek advice from a healthcare professional who can guide on the correct dosage.

- Consider adding powdered ashwagandha to your smoothies or taking it in capsule form.

- Utilize ginseng either through standardized supplements or traditional teas.

Minerals in Herbs: Horsetail and Nettle

Herbs such as horsetail and nettle provide essential minerals crucial for maintaining bone density. Horsetail is rich in silica, a mineral that contributes to the synthesis of collagen and cartilage, providing structural support to the bones. Nettle, abundant in calcium and magnesium, enhances bone strength and density, playing a preventive role against osteoporosis.

To maximize their benefits:

- Infuse horsetail tea or use horsetail supplements after consulting a healthcare practitioner.

- Include nettle in your diet via fresh leaves in soups or through dried leaf supplements.

Combining Herbal Supplements

The synergy between various herbal supplements can amplify their beneficial effects on bone health. Under the guidance of a healthcare provider, individuals can combine these herbs to create an optimal regimen that addresses multiple facets of osteoporosis. For instance, a combination of turmeric's anti-inflammatory properties and nettle's mineral content can provide comprehensive support.

To achieve this goal:

- Work closely with your healthcare provider to develop a personalized herbal supplement plan.

- Start with lower doses to assess tolerance and gradually increase based on professional advice.

- Monitor your bone density and overall health regularly to make necessary adjustments.

Holistic Approach and Lifestyle Integration

While herbal supplements offer promising results, incorporating them within a broader lifestyle strategy yields the best outcomes. Ensuring adequate calcium and vitamin D intake, alongside weight-bearing exercises, can dramatically boost the efficacy of herbal treatments (Mount Sinai Health System, n.d.). Regular physical activity not only increases bone mass but also improves coordination and balance, critical factors in preventing falls and fractures.

Research and Evidence

Empirical evidence supports the use of various herbal supplements in managing osteoporosis. Studies indicate that Traditional Chinese Medicine herbs like Herba epimedin, Fructus ligustri lucidi, and Fructus psoraleae have significant osteoblastic and anti-osteoclastic actions. Clinical trials reveal that these herbs protect and even enhance bone mineral density, especially in postmenopausal women (Leung et al., 2013).

Moreover, scientific data emphasizes that early and consistent use of natural remedies can prevent the decline in bone density often experienced with age and hormonal changes. For instance, research indicates that regular consumption of soy isoflavones helps maintain bone density in menopausal women, thanks to its phytoestrogen content. Meanwhile, herbs like Puerariae radix have shown positive effects on bone loss in both ovariectomized mice and castrated male mice, indicating their wide-ranging applicability (Cui et al., 2013).

Conclusion

By integrating herbal supplements like turmeric, Boswellia, ginseng, ashwagandha, horsetail, and nettle into a comprehensive healthcare plan, individuals can significantly enhance their bone health. Utilizing empirical evidence and professional guidance ensures that these natural remedies are both safe and effective. Remember, achieving the best results requires a balanced approach that includes proper diet, adequate exercise, and regular medical consultation.

As we navigate the complexities of osteoporosis treatment, it's clear that a holistic, evidence driven approach can harmonize personal well-being with broader societal benefits. This method ensures that while economic growth remains vital, human welfare rightfully takes precedence. Through careful consideration and adaptation of natural remedies, we empower ourselves towards better bone health and improved quality of life.

Importance of Vitamin D for Bone Strength

Vitamin D plays an essential role in bone health by aiding the body's absorption of calcium, which is critical for bone mineralization and density. Although sunlight is a natural source of vitamin D, relying solely on it may not be enough, particularly for individuals living in areas with limited sun exposure or those who spend most of their time indoors. This is where supplementation or consuming fortified foods becomes crucial.

Individuals with vitamin D deficiencies should consider integrating specific foods into their diets. Rich sources of vitamin D include fatty fish like salmon and trout, which also provide a range of other nutritional benefits. Adding eggs and fortified dairy products to your meals can further bolster your vitamin D intake. For example, many milk brands are fortified with vitamin D, providing a convenient way to ensure you're getting enough of this vital nutrient.

Regularly monitoring vitamin D levels is key to maintaining strong bones and preventing osteoporosis. It's advisable to consult with a healthcare provider for periodic blood tests to track your vitamin D status. By keeping tabs on these levels, you can adjust your intake accordingly, perhaps by increasing your consumption of vitamin D-rich foods or considering supplements if necessary. (Branch, 2023)

Another practical step is being mindful of the balance between sun exposure and skin protection.

While sunlight helps produce vitamin D, it's important to protect your skin to prevent harmful UV radiation effects. If you decide to spend more time outdoors, aim for short periods of sun exposure without sunscreen early in the morning or late in the afternoon, which can help without substantial risk of skin damage.

Here is what you can do to achieve optimal vitamin D levels:

- First, incorporate vitamin D-rich foods such as fatty fish, eggs, and fortified dairy products into your daily diet.

- Second, consider taking vitamin D supplements, especially during winter months or if you spend most of your time indoors.

- Third, monitor your vitamin D levels through regular check-ups with your healthcare provider.

- Fourth, balance sun exposure by spending short, safe periods outside without sunscreen.

Ensuring adequate vitamin D levels can complement other treatments and reinforce overall bone health. It works synergistically with calcium to fortify your skeletal system, reducing your risk of fractures and other complications associated with osteoporosis. During the course of various studies, vitamin D and calcium have shown promising results in improving bone mineral density (BMD) and reducing fracture incidences (Laird et al., 2010).

Speaking of calcium, it's another cornerstone of bone health. Our bodies need calcium to build and maintain strong bones, but we cannot produce it internally; it must come from our diet. Foods rich in calcium include dairy products like milk, cheese, and yogurt, as well as leafy green vegetables, tofu, and fortified juices and cereals. Dairy alternatives like almond, soy, and oat milk are also often fortified with calcium and can be excellent substitutes for those who are lactose intolerant or following a plant-based diet.

The interplay between calcium and vitamin D is crucial. Vitamin D enhances calcium absorption, ensuring that the calcium you consume is effectively used by your body. Together, they form a powerful duo in maintaining bone density and preventing osteoporosis. A deficiency in either nutrient can compromise bone health, leading to increased risks of fractures and other bone-related issues.

For adults, particularly those over 50, it is recommended to consume about 1,200 mg of calcium per day. Younger adults generally need around 1,000 mg daily. These requirements can often be met through a combination of diet and supplements. Consulting with a healthcare provider can help determine if you need additional supplements based on your dietary intake and lifestyle (Branch, 2023). Calcium citrate is shown to be more easily absorbed by the body. Also a chelated version of magnesium, like magnesium glyciuate is less likely to cause diarrhea.

Remember, while both vitamin D and calcium are fundamental to bone health, they are part of a broader approach to managing and treating osteoporosis. A balanced diet rich in essential nutrients, coupled with regular physical activity, particularly weight-bearing exercises like walking, jogging, or strength training, can significantly enhance bone density and overall health.

In conclusion, maintaining optimal levels of vitamin D and calcium is imperative for bone health and prevention of osteoporosis. By combining dietary sources, appropriate supplementation, and lifestyle adjustments, you can take proactive steps to safeguard your bone health. Regular medical check-ups will help keep your nutrient levels in check, allowing timely interventions if needed. Embracing these evidence-based practices ensures a robust foundation for healthier bones and a better quality of life.

Harnessing Natural Methods for Bone Health

Throughout this chapter, we have delved into the potential of various natural remedies in treating osteoporosis and improving bone density. By examining specific herbal supplements such as turmeric, Boswellia, ginseng, ashwagandha, horsetail, and nettle, we have highlighted their individual and synergistic benefits for bone health.

Returning to the initial premise, the exploration of natural remedies provides a promising alternative or complement to conventional treatments for osteoporosis. Our position aligns with a holistic approach that integrates these herbal supplements within a broader healthcare strategy. This includes maintaining an adequate intake of calcium and vitamin D, engaging in weightbearing exercises, and ensuring regular medical consultations.

It is important to remember, however, that not all natural remedies work the same way for everyone. The effectiveness of these herbs can vary based on individual health conditions, existing medications, and the body's unique response. Thus, it is essential for readers to consult healthcare professionals before starting any new supplement regimen. Personalizing treatment plans ensures safety and maximizes the potential benefits.

On a broader scale, the integration of natural remedies in osteoporosis management reflects a growing trend towards sustainable and preventive healthcare. It harmonizes economic considerations with personal well-being, aligning with a more inclusive model where traditional knowledge and modern science coexist. This comprehensive approach not only benefits individuals but also contributes positively to public health outcomes by reducing the burden of osteoporosis-related complications.

As you consider incorporating these natural remedies into your lifestyle, think about how they fit into your overall health strategy. Reflect on the balance between diet, exercise, and supplementation, making adjustments as needed under professional guidance. Osteoporosis management is a journey, and through informed choices, you can take proactive steps towards stronger bones and improved quality of life.

By embracing evidence-driven practices and maintaining a holistic perspective, you empower yourself to navigate the complexities of osteoporosis with confidence. Let this chapter serve as a guide and a springboard for further exploration, encouraging a thoughtful and balanced approach to enhancing your bone health naturally.

References

American Academy of Orthopedic Surgeons. (n.d.). *Vitamin D for Good Bone Health.*
Retrieved from https://orthoinfo.aaos.org/en/staying-healthy/vitamin-d-for-good-bone-health/

Leung, P.-C., & Siu, W.-S. (2013). *Herbal treatment for osteoporosis: A current review. Journal of Traditional and Complementary Medicine*, 2(3), 82.
https://doi.org/10.4103/22254110.110407

National Institute of Arthritis and Musculoskeletal and Skin Diseases. (2023). *Calcium and Vitamin D: Important for Bone Health.* Retrieved from
https://www.niams.nih.gov/healthtopics/calcium-and-vitamin-d-important-bone-health

Wang, Z., Li, J., Sun, Y., Yao, M., Gao, J., Yang, Z., Shi, Q., Cui, X., & Wang, Y. (2013). *Chinese Herbal Medicine for Osteoporosis: A Systematic Review of Randomized Controlled Trails. Evidence-based Complementary and Alternative Medicine : eCAM*, 2013.
https://doi.org/10.1155/2013/356260

Laird, E., Ward, M., McSorley, E., Strain, J. J., & Wallace, J. (2010). *Vitamin D and Bone*

Health; Potential Mechanisms. Nutrients, 2(7), 693. https://doi.org/10.3390/nu2070693

Mount Sinai Health System. (n.d.). *Osteoporosis*. https://www.mountsinai.org/healthlibrary/condition/osteoporosis

Chapter 3

Lifestyle Changes for Better Bone Health

Imagine waking up each day feeling stronger, more balanced, and full of vitality despite the steady march of time. Achieving this vision is not as far-fetched as it might seem, especially when you consider the significant impact that lifestyle choices can have on bone health. From the foods we consume to the activities we engage in, every decision plays a role in either fortifying or undermining our skeletal system. This chapter delves into the actionable steps you can take to naturally bolster your bones, offering a path toward a healthier, more resilient life.

Osteoporosis and declining bone density are increasingly common concerns as we age, but the true gravity of these conditions often goes unnoticed until a fracture occurs. Bones, much like other parts of our body, need continual maintenance and care. Unfortunately, modern habits— such as sedentary lifestyles, poor diet, and harmful substance use—can exacerbate bone deterioration. For instance, excessive alcohol consumption and smoking interfere with calcium absorption, weakening bones over time. Even certain popular carbonated drinks contribute to bone decay due to their high phosphoric acid content. The problem becomes even more pressing when considering the consequences: broken bones lead to reduced mobility, longer recovery times, and in severe cases, a dramatic shift in quality of life.

In this chapter, we will explore how specific lifestyle changes can become powerful tools in managing and even improving bone health. We'll dive into the benefits of regular weight-bearing exercises and resistance training, which stimulate bone formation and increase density. We'll also cover how nutrition plays a crucial role, highlighting key nutrients such as calcium, vitamin D, and magnesium that are essential for bone strength. Additionally, we'll discuss the importance of avoiding detrimental habits like smoking and excessive alcohol consumption, as well as practical strategies for integrating these adjustments into daily life. By understanding and applying these principles, you can take proactive steps to manage osteoporosis and enhance your overall well-being.

The Role of Exercise in Strengthening Bones

Engaging in weight-bearing exercises such as walking, jogging, or dancing is an excellent way to stimulate bone formation and strengthen your bones. You might be thinking, "Won't these activities just wear down my joints?" On the contrary, studies have demonstrated that the mechanical stress from weight-bearing exercises actually encourages the deposition of calcium in your bones, enhancing their density and strength. This kind of exercise essentially gives a wake-up call to your bone-forming cells, nudging them into action.

If you're wondering where to start, here are some practical steps you can take:

- Begin with low-impact activities like walking. If you're new to exercising, this is a gentle yet effective way to get your body accustomed to movement.

- Gradually introduce more dynamic exercises, like jogging or dancing, as your comfort and confidence grow. These higher-impact activities can further enhance the benefits for your bones.

- Aim for consistency rather than intensity. It's better to engage in moderate activity regularly than to exert yourself excessively on sporadic occasions.

Resistance training with weights or resistance bands is another crucial aspect of maintaining and improving bone health. This type of exercise not only boosts muscle strength but also supports bone density by applying targeted stress to various areas of your skeleton. You may hear "resistance training" and picture intense weightlifting sessions at the gym, but it doesn't have to be that daunting. Even simple exercises using your own body weight, free weights, or resistance bands can yield significant benefits.

To integrate resistance training into your routine:

- Start with lighter weights or resistance bands and gradually increase the load as you build strength.

- Focus on key muscle groups that surround and support your bones, such as those in your back, legs, and arms. Exercises like squats, lunges, and shoulder presses are particularly beneficial.

- Consider consulting with a physical therapist or a trainer who is experienced in working with individuals with osteoporosis. They can help you design a safe and effective program tailored to your needs.

Regular engagement in weight-bearing exercises and resistance training can maintain and even increase bone density, thereby reducing the risk of fractures—a concern that becomes more pronounced as we age. It's never too late to start incorporating these practices into your lifestyle, and the benefits extend far beyond bone health. Improved muscle strength, better balance, and enhanced overall well-being are just a few of the additional perks you'll gain.

Consistency is key when it comes to reaping the full rewards of these exercises. Think of bone health as a long-term investment. Just as compound interest accumulates over time, so do the benefits of regular exercise. Set realistic goals and remember that every step counts—literally.

Incorporating varied weight-bearing activities into your routine can target different areas of the body, contributing to overall bone strength. Much like a diversified investment portfolio, a variety of exercises ensures that no part of your body is neglected. Walking primarily benefits the bones in your legs, hips, and lower spine, but adding upper body exercises like push-ups or rowing can provide comprehensive support to your skeletal system.

Imagine giving your bones a holistic workout:

- Mix in different types of weight-bearing activities throughout the week. For instance, walk on Mondays, jog on Wednesdays, and dance on Fridays.

- Add activities that challenge your balance and stability, such as tai chi or yoga. These not only improve bone strength but also reduce the risk of falls.

- Ensure that your routine includes both high-impact and low-impact exercises to cater to all parts of your body.

Variety keeps things interesting and motivates you to stick with your exercise regimen, making it easier to sustain the benefits for bone health over the long run.

While we emphasize physical activity, it's essential to approach exercise safely, especially if you have osteoporosis. Consult with your healthcare provider before starting any new exercise routine. They may suggest tests such as a bone density measurement or fitness assessment to guide your exercise choices. Tailoring your activities based on medical advice ensures that you're protecting your bones while strengthening them (Mayo Clinic, 2023).

The effectiveness of physical exercise on bone health also depends on the quality and intensity of the workouts. According to recent findings, reaching the mechanical intensity needed to generate significant ground reaction force is crucial. This means that simply walking might not be sufficient to improve bone mass, although it does help limit its progressive loss. Activities like stair climbing, volleyball, and Tai Chi have shown greater benefits because they hit the mark in terms of load intensity (Benedetti et al., 2018).

Combining different forms of exercise—such as aerobic, strength, resistance, balance, and flexibility exercises—within a single routine can amplify the benefits, especially for those who might find it challenging to stick to one type of exercise. Programs that integrate these elements can potentially offer a comprehensive approach to bone health, addressing multiple facets of strength, stability, and endurance.

On a more advanced note, whole body vibration (WBV) exercises are emerging as a promising option. These involve the use of specialized equipment to produce vibrations that stimulate muscle contractions. Some research indicates that WBV can effectively improve muscle strength and balance, which are critical for fall prevention. However, the impact of WBV on actual bone density remains somewhat controversial, and anyone considering this should do so under professional guidance, especially given the contraindications often associated with older age (Benedetti et al., 2018).

Ultimately, the intersection of individual freedom and social responsibility plays a pivotal role in how we approach policy changes related to public health issues like osteoporosis. Encouraging accessible, evidence-based exercise programs and promoting education about bone health can empower individuals to take charge of their well-being. At the same time, ensuring that policies are in place to provide support and resources for those who need them most exemplifies the balance between personal responsibility and collective welfare.

By weaving these scientifically backed strategies into your daily life, you're taking important steps toward not only managing osteoporosis but also enhancing your quality of life. Remember, healthy bones are the foundation for a robust, active, and independent lifestyle.

Adopting a Bone-Friendly Lifestyle

Managing osteoporosis naturally involves making lifestyle adjustments that can significantly impact bone health. Avoiding certain habits and ensuring adequate nutrient intake are essential steps to maintain strong bones and prevent further deterioration. Let's dive deeper into practical actions you can take, supported by empirical evidence.

First off, it's crucial to avoid excessive consumption of alcohol and tobacco. These substances interfere with calcium absorption, which is detrimental to bone strength. Research has shown that smoking reduces bone mass and increases the risk of fractures (Chen et al., 2020). Additionally, alcohol can lead to bone loss due to its effect on osteoblasts, the cells responsible for bone formation. If you are a smoker or frequently consume alcohol, consider these steps to reduce your intake:

- **Seek Professional Help:** Consult with healthcare providers for resources on quitting smoking and reducing alcohol consumption.

- **Replace Habits:** Find healthier activities to replace smoking or drinking, such as exercising or engaging in a hobby.

- **Support Systems:** Join support groups that focus on cessation programs for both smoking and alcohol consumption.

Next, it's advisable to limit the intake of carbonated beverages high in phosphoric acid. While moderate intake may not harm bone density significantly (Barrett-Connor et al., 1997), excessive consumption can leach calcium from bones, leading to weaker bone structure. Phosphoric acid in cola drinks, for example, has been linked to reduced bone mineral density and an increased risk of fractures.

Here's how to manage your intake of carbonated beverages:

- **Read Labels Carefully:** Look for drinks low in phosphoric acid or choose alternatives like water, herbal teas, or freshly squeezed juices.

- **Moderation is Key:** If you enjoy carbonated beverages, try to limit their consumption to occasional treats rather than daily indulgence.

- **Increase Calcium-Rich Foods:** Balance your intake by consuming foods rich in calcium alongside any carbonated drinks you do consume.

Ensuring adequate intake of essential nutrients like calcium, vitamin D, and magnesium is another cornerstone of supporting bone health. Calcium is fundamental for bone strength, while vitamin D enhances calcium absorption. Magnesium plays a crucial role in bone formation and the structural development of bones. Here are steps to ensure you're getting enough of these vital nutrients:

- **Calcium Sources:** Include dairy products like milk, cheese, and yogurt. Leafy green vegetables, almonds, and fortified plant-based milks are also excellent sources.

- **Vitamin D Through Sunlight:** Spend some time outdoors every day to let your skin synthesize vitamin D from sunlight. Alternatively, consider vitamin D supplements, especially during the winter months or if you live in areas with limited sunlight.

- **Magnesium-Rich Foods:** Incorporate nuts, seeds, whole grains, and legumes into your diet to boost magnesium levels.

Maintaining a healthy body weight is critical to reduce strain on bones and lower the risk of fractures. Both underweight and overweight conditions can negatively impact bone health. Being underweight may lead to bone loss and fractures, while being overweight increases the load on bones, especially those in the lower body, increasing fracture risk. To keep your body weight within a healthy range, consider these guidelines:

- **Balanced Diet:** Follow a diet rich in fruits, vegetables, lean proteins, and whole grains to maintain an optimal weight.

- **Regular Exercise:** Engage in weight-bearing exercises such as walking, jogging, or resistance training to strengthen bones and muscles. Exercise helps improve balance and coordination, reducing the risk of falls and fractures.

- **Monitor Weight Regularly:** Keep track of your weight through regular check-ins. If you notice significant changes, consult a healthcare provider for appropriate interventions.

- **Avoid Extreme Diets:** Steer clear of fad diets that promise quick weight loss but lack essential nutrients. Focus on sustainable eating habits that provide the necessary nutrients for overall health and bone strength.

Adopting these bone-friendly habits can significantly safeguard and enhance your bone health. It's important to take a holistic view, balancing lifestyle choices with nutritional intake to manage osteoporosis effectively. By avoiding harmful substances, limiting unhealthy beverage consumption, ensuring sufficient nutrient intake, and maintaining a healthy weight, you can create a robust defense against bone weakness and fractures.

In summary, practical lifestyle adjustments can play a pivotal role in managing osteoporosis and improving bone health. Steering clear of excessive alcohol and tobacco, moderating carbonated beverage consumption, prioritizing essential nutrients, and keeping a healthy weight are all actionable steps that can make a significant difference. Remember, your personal responsibility is key, but so is accessing the right support and information. Engaging with healthcare professionals and utilizing available resources will help you navigate these changes smoothly and effectively. Stay proactive, stay informed, and keep moving towards better bone health.

Taking Control of Your Bone Health

As we have explored in this chapter, making lifestyle adjustments can significantly impact bone health and naturally manage osteoporosis. The role of exercise in strengthening bones is paramount. Weight-bearing exercises and resistance training are effective strategies to enhance bone density and prevent fractures. Engaging in activities like walking, jogging, dancing, and using resistance bands or weights helps activate your bone-forming cells and build stronger bones. This approach requires consistency and variety in your routine to provide comprehensive support to your skeletal system.

Reflecting on our initial discussion, it's clear that managing osteoporosis involves more than just physical activity. Avoiding habits like excessive alcohol consumption and smoking is crucial, as these can impede calcium absorption and compromise bone health. Additionally, moderating the intake of carbonated beverages that contain phosphoric acid can further protect your bones.

Our current stance underscores the importance of ensuring adequate nutrient intake. Foods rich in calcium, vitamin D, and magnesium contribute to maintaining strong bones. A balanced diet that includes dairy products, leafy greens, nuts, and seeds supports bone formation and maintenance. Coupled with regular, weight-bearing exercise, this holistic approach forms a robust defense against osteoporosis.

However, some readers might be concerned about starting an exercise regimen, especially if they have not been active for a while. It's important to consult healthcare providers before beginning any new physical activities. Tailoring your exercise plan based on medical advice ensures safety while maximizing the benefits.

On a wider scale, adopting a bone-friendly lifestyle can lead to improved public health outcomes. Policies that promote accessible exercise programs and education on bone health can empower individuals to take proactive steps toward better well-being. Encouraging healthy habits within communities fosters a collective responsibility to support one another in managing conditions like osteoporosis.

In closing, managing osteoporosis through lifestyle adjustments is both achievable and beneficial. By incorporating exercise, avoiding harmful habits, ensuring nutrient intake, and maintaining a healthy weight, you can significantly enhance your bone health. This journey requires dedication and support, but the rewards—a robust, active, and independent life—are well worth the effort. As you continue this path, remember that every positive change contributes to your overall health and longevity. Keep striving towards a healthier, stronger future.

References

Mayo Clinic. (2023). *Exercising with osteoporosis: Stay active the safe way. Mayo Clinic.* Retrieved from https://www.mayoclinic.org/diseases-conditions/osteoporosis/indepth/osteoporosis/art-20044989

Harvard Health. (2021). *Slowing bone loss with weight-bearing exercise. Staying Healthy.* Retrieved from https://www.health.harvard.edu/staying-healthy/slowing-bone-loss-with-weightbearing-exercise

Benedetti, M. G., Furlini, G., Zati, A., Mauro, G. L. (2018). *The effectiveness of physical exercise on bone density in osteoporotic patients. BioMed Research International*, 2018, 4840531. https://doi.org/10.1155/2018/4840531

Kim, S. H., Morton, D. J., & Barrett-Connor, E. L. (1997). *Carbonated beverage consumption and bone mineral density among older women: the Rancho Bernardo Study.* American Journal of Public Health, *87*(2), 276. https://doi.org/10.2105/ajph.87.2.276

Chen, L., Liu, R., Zhao, Y., & Shi, Z. (2020). *High consumption of soft drinks is associated with an increased risk of fracture: A 7-year follow-up study. Nutrients*, 12(2), 530. https://doi.org/10.3390/nu12020530

Chapter 4

Dietary Guidelines for Strong Bones

Imagine your bones as the sturdy framework of a well-constructed building. Just like any structure needs quality materials to maintain its integrity, your bones require essential nutrients to stay strong and prevent conditions like osteoporosis. Recognizing the critical role nutrition plays in bone health is the first step towards a life where fractures and bone density issues are rare occurrences rather than common concerns.

The primary problem stands clear: without adequate nutrition, our bones suffer. For example, calcium deficiency can lead to brittle bones that break easily under minor stress. Vitamin D, crucial for calcium absorption, often gets overlooked despite being vital for bone strength. Magnesium, another key player in bone formation, helps optimize calcium's role, yet many diets fall short of this mineral. Moreover, omega-3 fatty acids provide anti-inflammatory benefits that indirectly support bone health, while zinc and Vitamin K contribute to bone tissue growth and regulation. When these nutrients are missing or imbalanced in our diet, our skeletal system becomes vulnerable to deterioration and disease.

Studies have shown that magnesium should be taken separately from calcium. It is best taken at night since it relaxes the muscles and helps with sleep. Try to buy organic when possible. Watch out for sugar content as well.

This chapter dives deeply into the dietary recommendations necessary to enhance your bone health and ward off osteoporosis. It explores the importance of incorporating nutrient-rich foods like dairy products, leafy greens, fatty fish, nuts, seeds, and fortified cereals into your meals. You will also learn practical tips on ensuring sufficient intake of calcium, Vitamin D, magnesium, and other essential nutrients through everyday foods. By the end of this chapter, you'll have a comprehensive understanding of how to build a meal plan that supports robust bones, aiming to equip you with actionable steps toward a healthier, more resilient skeletal system.

Importance of Essential Nutrients

Nutrient-rich foods are like the foundation on which we build strong bones. To maintain optimal bone health, certain key nutrients are indispensable, and ensuring that they make their way into our daily diet is critical. Let's explore some of these essential elements and the delicious foods that carry them.

Calcium ranks high when discussing bone health, as it is the primary building block of bone tissue. Delicious and abundant sources include dairy products like milk, yogurt, and cheese. Remember to consume low-fat or fat-free versions if you're watching your calorie intake. If dairy isn't a part of your diet, fear not - leafy greens such as kale, broccoli, and Bok Choy are excellent alternatives. Additionally, many cereals today come fortified with calcium, making breakfast a delightful opportunity to bolster your bone strength.

Here's what you can do to ensure sufficient calcium intake:

- Incorporate dairy products like milk, yogurt, or cheese into your meals.

- Add leafy greens to your dishes; think spinach in your omelet or kale in your salad. Try to buy these types of vegetables. Organic of course, Spinach and kale are very good for you, but they can harbor chemicals if you do not buy organic.

  - Choose cereals and plant-based milks (like almond or soy) that are fortified with calcium.

While calcium is crucial, its effectiveness heavily relies on Vitamin D, often dubbed the "sunshine vitamin." This nutrient enhances the absorption of calcium into the bloodstream. Sunlight exposure is a primary natural source, but foods fortified with Vitamin D, such as orange juice and cereal, can also help. Fatty fishlike salmon and mackerel are particularly rich in these nutrients, offering an added bonus of heart-healthy omega-3 fatty acids.

Turning our attention to magnesium, it's clear this mineral plays a pivotal role in not just bone formation but also in over 300 biochemical reactions in the body. Nuts and seeds are fantastic sources - consider snacking on almonds, cashews, or pumpkin seeds. Whole grains can also up your magnesium game. The synergy between calcium and magnesium creates stronger bones, with magnesium aiding in calcium absorption and promoting bone mineralization.

To maximize magnesium benefits:

  - Eat a handful of nuts or seeds as a snack or add them to your salads and yogurts.

  - opt for whole grain versions of bread, pasta, and rice.

  - Consider incorporating legumes like black beans or chickpeas into your meals. Again try to get your vegetables from Organic sources.

The power of nutrients doesn't stop there. Omega-3 fatty acids, which reduce inflammation and support bone density, are another

•

group of superheroes deserving our attention. Fatty fish such as salmon, sardines, and mackerel are rich in these essential fats. For those who prefer plant-based options, flaxseeds and chia seeds are excellent choices. These tiny seeds can be sprinkled over oatmeal, blended into smoothies, or even mixed into baked goods, making it easy to boost your omega-3 intake.

When aiming to get more omega-3s:

- Include fatty fish in your meal plan a couple of times a week.

- Add ground flaxseeds or chia seeds to your breakfast cereal or smoothies.

- Use walnut oil or canola oil for cooking and salad dressings.

Zinc and Vitamin K are lesser known yet equally vital players in the realm of bone health. Zinc supports bone tissue growth and repair, while <u>Vitamin K is crucial</u> for bone mineralization and the regulation of calcium in the blood. Foods that deliver these nutrients include meats such as beef and chicken, and vegetarian-friendly options like beans and lentils. Broccoli and Brussels sprouts pack a punch with Vitamin K, making them not only tasty but beneficial for your bones.

Vitamin K2 activates Osteocalcin, a protein produced by Osteoblasts. It can help calcium to bind to your bones.

To ensure you're getting enough zinc and Vitamin K:

Incorporate lean meats and beans into your meals.

- Enjoy broccoli or Brussels sprouts steamed, roasted, or raw in a salad.

- Look for fortified foods that provide additional zinc and vitamin K.

As you might notice, consuming a diverse range of nutrient-rich foods isn't just about ticking off boxes on a nutritional checklist – it's about creating a holistic approach to diet that naturally includes essential vitamins and minerals. By consistently incorporating these dietary recommendations, you lay the groundwork for stronger bones and overall better health.

Approaching your diet with variety ensures that you're covering all bases. Not only do these foods contribute to bone health, but they also bring other health benefits, such as improved digestion, enhanced immune function, and reduced chronic disease risk. Each bite taken with intention towards bone health compounds, leading to a sturdier skeletal system capable of supporting you through life's many adventures.

Let's understand that the balance between economic interests and human welfare extends even to our dietary choices. While choosing fresh and organic options may sometimes be pricier, investing in quality nutrition pays off in the long run, much like how balanced policies benefit society. Advocating for affordable, nutritious food aligns with our broader goals of handing more power to people, ensuring everyone has access to the essentials needed for a healthy life.

Moreover, individual responsibility paired with societal support systems forms the bedrock of sustainable health practices. It's about taking charge of your dietary habits while advocating for community resources, education, and access to nutritious options. Together, we can create an environment where informed choices lead to healthier, stronger communities.

Incorporating these practical dietary guidelines can transform how we approach bone health. It's not just about reacting to osteoporosis or bone density problems but proactively strengthening our foundation. Balanced nutrition rooted in empirical evidence ensures we are empowered with knowledge to make smarter decisions. Here's to healthier bones and a healthier future, achieved one nutrient-packed meal at a time.

Benefits of Anti-inflammatory Foods

Foods like berries, fatty fish, and green tea contain antioxidants that combat inflammation and protect bone cells. These foods aren't just delicious additions to your diet; they're powerful allies in the fight against inflammation and bone degeneration. Antioxidants help neutralize free radicals—those erratic molecules that can cause cellular damage—and thus play a crucial role in maintaining healthy bones.

To get the most out of these anti-inflammatory benefits, consider incorporating the following into your meals:

- **Berries**: Blueberries, strawberries, blackberries, and raspberries are packed with vitamins, minerals, and particularly antioxidants. Make it a habit to add a handful of mixed berries to your morning yogurt or oatmeal. Alternatively, you could enjoy them as a mid-day snack. All Organic due to pesticides in the foods.

- **Fatty Fish**: Salmon, mackerel, and sardines provide not just Omega-3 fatty acids, but also important nutrients like Vitamin D, which is vital for calcium absorption. Aim to include fatty fish in your diet at least twice a week. Grilling or baking fish is a good way to retain its nutritional value without adding unwanted fats.

- **Green Tea**: Rich in catechins, a type of antioxidant, green tea offers multiple health benefits, including bone protection. Swap your cup of coffee with a soothing cup of green tea. Upgrading to matcha—a form of powdered green tea—can offer even more concentrated benefits.

Including turmeric and ginger in meals can help reduce inflammation and promote bone healing. Both are rooted deeply in traditional medicine and have been shown in modern studies to possess strong anti-inflammatory properties. They can be easily added to a variety of dishes, enhancing both flavor and health benefits.

Here is what you can do to incorporate these spices effectively:

- **Turmeric**: This golden spice can be sprinkled into soups, stews, and curries. Turmeric latte is another exciting way to savor its benefits. Simply mix a teaspoon of turmeric powder into warm milk, add a dash of black pepper to aid absorption, and sweeten with a bit of honey if desired.

- **Ginger**: Fresh ginger root enhances both savory and sweet dishes. You can grate fresh ginger into stir-fries, marinades, and salad dressings. Ginger tea is a comforting alternative, especially during colder seasons; simply slice some fresh ginger and steep it in hot water.

Consuming a plant-based diet rich in fruits, vegetables, and whole grains can lower inflammation levels and support bone density. Evidence consistently shows that diets high in plant-based foods offer numerous health benefits, including enhanced bone health. Whole grains, fruits, and vegetables are not only brimming with essential vitamins and minerals but also packed with fiber that supports overall health.

To transition smoothly to a more plant-based diet, try these steps:

- Start by filling half of your plate with vegetables at each meal. Leafy greens like spinach, kale, and broccoli are especially beneficial due to their high calcium content. •
Replace refined grains with whole grains such as quinoa, brown rice, and whole wheat. These grains provide more nutrients and fiber compared to their refined counterparts.

Incorporate more legumes like lentils, chickpeas, and beans into your diet. They're excellent sources of protein and other nutrients necessary for maintaining bone health.

- Experiment with meatless meals several times a week. Think about plant-based proteins like tofu, tempeh, and seitan as main components in your recipes.

Avoiding processed foods and excessive sugar intake can prevent inflammation and preserve bone health. Processed foods often contain trans fats, high levels of sodium, and added sugars, all of which contribute to chronic inflammation and, subsequently, bone deterioration.

To keep these harmful elements in check:

- Prioritize home-cooked meals over pre-packaged foods. Preparing meals from scratch allows you complete control over ingredients, ensuring they align with your health goals.
- Read labels meticulously when grocery shopping. Look out for high levels of salt, sugar, and artificial ingredients, opting instead for items with natural and minimal ingredient lists.

- Replace sugary snacks with healthier alternatives. Fresh fruit, nuts, and yogurt are great choices that won't spike your blood sugar levels and will provide sustained energy throughout the day.

- Limit the intake of sugary beverages. Soda, energy drinks, and even fruit juices can be loaded with hidden sugars. Opt for water or herbal tea as a healthier option.

In summary, prioritizing anti-inflammatory foods can reduce the risk of bone-related conditions and enhance overall well-being. The evidence is clear: a diet rich in anti-inflammatory, nutrientdense foods can significantly boost bone health. Berries, fatty fish, and green tea act as formidable warriors against oxidative stress, while turmeric and ginger work seamlessly to tackle inflammation head-on. A shift towards plant-based eating further cements this foundation, lowering inflammation levels naturally and promoting robust bone density. On the flip side, stepping away from processed foods and curbing sugar intake can stave off harmful inflammation, preserving bone health for the long term.

Ultimately, achieving and maintaining bone health isn't about restrictive dieting or making drastic changes overnight. It's about integrating these small, manageable adjustments into your daily routine to support your bones and overall health gradually and sustainably. Armed with this knowledge and a bit of effort, you can take proactive steps toward fortifying your bone health and living a vibrant, balanced life.

Impact of Hydration on Bone Health

Staying adequately hydrated is crucial for maintaining good bone health. When you think of strong bones, water might not be the first thing that comes to mind, but it's essential. Hydration supports proper mineralization and helps maintain a solid bone structure. Here's what this means in more practical terms: your bones are made up of minerals like calcium and phosphate, and these need to be continuously deposited and maintained within the bone matrix. Water plays a key role in this process by ensuring that these minerals are correctly transported and absorbed where they're needed most.

So, how can you make sure you're staying hydrated to support your bones?

- Keep a reusable water bottle with you and take small sips throughout the day.

- Pay attention to your body's signals, such as feeling thirsty or having dry mouth.

- Increase your water intake during hot weather or when you are physically active.

By incorporating these habits into your daily routine, you can help ensure that your bones receive the minerals they need to stay strong and healthy.

Water facilitates the transport of nutrients to bone cells, promoting their growth and repair. Picture a bustling highway, with nutrients as vehicles traveling to their destination—your bone cells. Being well-hydrated keeps these highways clear and efficient. It ensures that necessary nutrients aren't delayed in transit, allowing your bones to recover and rebuild effectively after any wear and tear. This all happens silently within your body, yet it's an integral part of maintaining robust bone health.

Dehydration, on the other hand, can have serious consequences for your bones. When you don't drink enough water, the efficiency of nutrient transportation diminishes. Over time, this can lead to weakened bones and a decrease in bone density. Think of it as trying to build a house without sufficient materials—it just won't stand strong. The same goes for your bones; lacking the necessary nutrients will impair their ability to fortify themselves, making them fragile and more prone to issues like osteoporosis.

Consuming water-rich foods, such as fruits and vegetables, is another excellent way to keep your hydration levels in check and support bone health. Fruits like cucumbers, watermelon, and strawberries are not only delicious but also packed with water. Vegetables such as celery, lettuce, and zucchini contribute significantly to your daily hydration needs while providing essential vitamins and minerals that benefit your bones.

Here's how you can incorporate more water-rich foods into your diet:

- Start your day with a fruit smoothie that includes high-water-content fruits like berries, melons, and citrus.

- Add salads loaded with hydrating vegetables like cucumber, bell peppers, and leafy greens to your meals.

- Snack on fresh fruit instead of processed options.

These small dietary adjustments can go a long way in keeping you hydrated and supporting your overall bone health.

Maintaining optimal hydration levels is crucial for supporting bone strength and preventing osteoporosis. It's easy to overlook the importance of drinking enough water, but its impact on our skeletal system is profound. By understanding how hydration works at a cellular level, we can make simple yet effective changes to our daily habits that ensure our bones remain strong and resilient throughout our lives.

In summary, ensuring adequate hydration involves a multi-faceted approach. Firstly, drinking water regularly and attentively is fundamental. Keep track of your water intake and aim to meet your daily needs, adjusting based on factors such as activity level and environmental conditions. Secondly, consuming water-rich foods provides an additional source of hydration, aiding in the continuous supply of water to your cells and tissues.

Lastly, being aware of the signs of dehydration can help you take proactive measures before it negatively impacts your bones. Signs such as dark urine, dry skin, and fatigue are indicators that it's time to increase your water intake. Staying vigilant about these signs can prevent long-term damage and support your bone health effectively.

These insights shed light on the often-overlooked connection between hydration and bone health. By making hydration a priority, you support not only your overall health but also the strength and resilience of your bones. Remember, simple changes in your daily routine can make a big difference. Embrace the power of water, both in your glass and on your plate, and give your bones the support they deserve.

Balancing Acidic and Alkaline Foods

Consuming too many acidic foods like meat and processed foods can lead to calcium loss from bones. When our diets are overly acidic, the body may pull calcium from our bones to neutralize the excess acid. This calcium depletion weakens bones over time and increases the risk of osteoporosis. It's important to be aware of the potential impact that a diet high in acidic foods can have on bone health.

On the other hand, alkaline foods such as fruits, vegetables, and nuts help neutralize acid levels in the body and support bone health. Alkaline foods contribute to a more balanced pH level, which can prevent the body from needing to use calcium reserves from bones. Here is what you can do in order to achieve the goal:

- Include a variety of fresh fruits and vegetables in your daily meals. Leafy greens, berries, citrus fruits, and root vegetables are particularly beneficial.

- Incorporate nuts and seeds into your snacks or meals. Almonds, chia seeds, and flaxseeds are excellent choices.

- Opt for plant-based protein sources, such as beans, lentils, and tofu, to balance the acidity from animal proteins.

Maintaining a diet that includes a balance of acidic and alkaline foods can promote bone density and reduce bone resorption. Balance is key here. While it's not necessary to eliminate acidic foods altogether, integrating more alkaline foods into your diet can create a healthier environment for your bones. Striking this balance might seem challenging at first, but it's quite manageable with some thoughtful planning.

Monitoring pH levels through diet can help prevent bone weakening and maintain bone mineral density. Some may find it helpful to keep track of their dietary intake and even measure their urinary pH levels periodically to ensure they are maintaining a good balance. Here are some tips to help manage your diet for optimal pH balance:

- Focus on eating whole, unprocessed foods. These tend to be less acidic and more nutrient-dense.

- Stay hydrated by drinking plenty of water throughout the day. Water is neutral and can help wash out excess acids.

- Be mindful of portion sizes. Consuming a small quantity of acidic foods won't harm your bones as long as it's balanced with a significant amount of alkaline food.

By adopting these practices, you can make a positive impact on your bone health. Understanding the interaction between diet and bone density underscores the importance of making informed choices about what we eat. Personal responsibility plays a significant role here; each decision made at the grocery store or dining table has the potential to either support or undermine our bone health.

To further understand the practical applications of these dietary choices, consider how a typical day's meals could look. Breakfast could start with a smoothie packed with leafy greens, berries, and almond milk. Lunch might include a colorful salad with a variety of vegetables and a handful of nuts. Dinner could feature grilled vegetables alongside a lean protein source like fish or tofu, finished with a dessert of fresh fruit.

It's not just about avoiding certain foods but rather embracing a varied and balanced diet. This approach aligns with both evidence-driven reasoning and personal freedom. You have the liberty to choose from an array of delicious and nourishing foods while ensuring that your choices support your overall health.

When government and corporate policies align to promote healthier food options, they help facilitate these important individual choices. Whether through subsidies for fresh produce or regulations on highly processed foods, such measures can help guide the population toward better nutritional habits without infringing on personal freedom. However, checks and balances are crucial to ensure these policies truly serve public interests rather than corporate profits alone.

In conclusion, striking a balance between acidic and alkaline foods is essential for preserving bone health and reducing the risk of osteoporosis. By focusing on consuming more fruits, vegetables, and nuts, while moderating meat and processed foods, you can help maintain bone density over time. Making small, consistent changes in your diet can result in significant longterm benefits for your bones. Embrace the power of your dietary choices, armed with evidence and a balanced approach, to enhance your overall well-being.

Remember, the path to better bone health doesn't have to be daunting. With each meal, you have the opportunity to invest in your future strength and vitality. So, relish in the journey towards stronger bones with optimism and confidence, knowing that you are making informed decisions based on sound evidence and a commitment to your welfare. By keeping a balanced perspective on your diet, you'll be well on your way to achieving robust bone health and preventing osteoporosis naturally and effectively.

Ensuring Lifelong Bone Health

As we have delved into specific dietary recommendations that can significantly enhance bone health and help prevent osteoporosis, it becomes clear that a well-rounded nutritional approach is paramount. Throughout this chapter, we've explored the essential nutrients necessary for strong bones, such as calcium, Vitamin D, magnesium, and omega-3 fatty acids, as well as the importance of hydration and balancing acidic and alkaline foods.

Reflecting on earlier points, one might recall the initial emphasis on nutrient-rich foods forming the foundation of bone health. This foundation is crucial because incorporating a variety of these nutrients into one's diet supports not only the structure but also the resilience of our bones. Our current stance is that achieving balanced nutrition through diverse and thoughtful food choices will considerably fortify bone health.

However, a concern for some readers may be the complexity of integrating these recommendations into daily life, especially amid busy schedules and varying access to highquality foods. It is essential to recognize that making small, gradual changes can lead to substantial improvements in bone health over time. For example, swapping out processed snacks for nuts or adding leafy greens to meals can make a significant difference without overwhelming the individual.

On a broader scale, the consequences of adopting these dietary changes could extend beyond personal health. When more people embrace diets rich in essential nutrients, societal benefits such as reduced healthcare costs related to osteoporosis and improved overall public health could follow. This aligns with the idea that individual responsibility coupled with systemic support can create healthier communities.

As we conclude this chapter, consider how powerful simple dietary adjustments can be in shaping your future health. By thoughtfully choosing nutrient-dense foods, you are laying the groundwork for stronger bones and a more resilient you. The journey towards optimal bone health is ongoing and filled with opportunities to learn and adapt. Remember, each meal is a step towards a more fortified skeletal system, poised to support you through all of life's adventures.

Embrace this journey with an informed mindset, and let small, consistent choices pave the way to a healthier future.

Chapter 5
Supplements for Bone Density

Maintaining healthy bones is crucial for overall well-being, especially as we age. Whether it's keeping up with grandchildren or pursuing a long-loved hobby, strong bones can make a significant difference in your quality of life. Supplements have increasingly gained attention for their role in supporting bone density and health. But how effective are these supplements, and what should you consider before starting them? Understanding the science and practicality behind various supplements can help you make more informed decisions about your bone health.

Osteoporosis and other bone density issues affect millions of adults worldwide, leading to fractures, mobility problems, and chronic pain. Our bones naturally lose density over time, particularly after menopause in women and later stages of life in men. Calcium deficiency is one major contributor, as our bodies rely on stored calcium in bones when dietary intake falls short. This can lead to weakened bones and increased fracture risk. Furthermore, inadequate levels of Vitamin D hinder calcium absorption, rendering calcium supplements less effective. Similarly, insufficient magnesium disrupts the balance necessary for optimal bone strength. Without addressing these key nutrients, managing bone health becomes significantly more challenging.

In this chapter, we'll explore various supplements that play a critical role in boosting bone density and maintaining overall bone health. From the essential minerals like calcium and magnesium to vitamins such as Vitamin D, we'll delve into how each one contributes uniquely to strengthening bones. You'll also learn practical steps on how to incorporate these supplements into your daily routine, including recommended dosages and food sources. Additionally, we'll discuss collagen's role in bone integrity and repair—a factor often overlooked but highly beneficial. By the end of this chapter, you'll be equipped with comprehensive knowledge to create a robust supplement strategy tailored to your needs, paving the way for healthier, stronger bones.

Key Supplements for Osteoporosis Management

When it comes to managing osteoporosis, taking the right supplements can be a game-changer. Let's dive into some key elements that could significantly boost your bone density and overall bone health.

First off, calcium is indispensable for maintaining bone strength and density. Our bones act as a reservoir of calcium; when the body's supply runs low, it pulls from this reserve, weakening the bones over time. This is why supplementing your diet with calcium is crucial, especially if you're prone to or already battling osteoporosis. Here's what you can do in order to ensure you get enough calcium:

- Incorporate calcium-rich foods like dairy products, leafy greens, and fortified cereals into your meals.

-

  If dietary intake is insufficient, opt for calcium supplements. Over-the-counter options abound, but making an informed choice is vital.

- Aim for around 1,000 to 1,200 milligrams of calcium daily, depending on your age and specific needs.

Adding to the mix, Vitamin D is another essential component. Without adequate Vitamin D, your body struggles to absorb calcium efficiently, rendering those calcium supplements less effective. Think of Vitamin D as the gatekeeper—without it, calcium can't get through to where it's needed most. For optimal bone density, here are some steps to bolster your Vitamin D intake:

- Spend a bit more time in the sun, as sunlight is a natural source of Vitamin D.

- Include foods rich in Vitamin D such as fatty fish, egg yolks, and fortified foods in your daily diet.

- Consider a daily Vitamin D supplement, especially during the winter months or if you live in a region with limited sunlight. Consult with your healthcare provider to determine the ideal dosage for you.

Next up is magnesium. Often overshadowed by calcium and Vitamin D, magnesium plays a critical role in bone formation and density. A good balance of calcium and magnesium ensures that each mineral works effectively. Magnesium helps convert Vitamin D into its active form, which then facilitates calcium absorption. Here's how you can make sure you're getting enough magnesium:

- Eat a variety of magnesium-rich foods, including nuts, seeds, whole grains, and dark leafy vegetables.

- If necessary, introduce a magnesium supplement into your routine.

- Balance is key—too much calcium without sufficient magnesium can lead to imbalances that compromise bone health.

Collagen should not be overlooked either. While not commonly associated with bone health, collagen provides structural integrity to bones and aids in the repair process. Collagen supplements contain amino acids that stimulate the production of proteins needed for bone fortification. For comprehensive bone health support, consider these methods:

- Include collagen-boosting foods like bone broth, chicken skin, fish, and egg whites in your diet.

- Opt for collagen supplements, especially if dietary sources are scarce. Look for hydrolyzed collagen, as it's easier for the body to absorb.

  Combining collagen supplements with other bone-supportive nutrients like Vitamin C can enhance their effectiveness.

Each of these supplements—calcium, Vitamin D, magnesium, and collagen—contributes uniquely to bone health. By integrating them thoughtfully, you can create a robust strategy to manage osteoporosis and improve bone density. Regular and consistent intake is key; skipping doses may diminish their benefits, so staying committed is crucial.

But remember, personal responsibility doesn't mean you need to shoulder this alone. Consult with your healthcare provider before starting any new supplement regimen. Their insights, grounded in empirical evidence, can help tailor a plan specific to your needs, ensuring that these supplements work harmoniously with any treatments you may already be undergoing.

By focusing not just on economic feasibility but also on tangible health outcomes, you bridge the gap between empirical data and personal well-being. You take proactive steps towards better bone health while contributing to a larger framework of public health improvement. The journey to better bone health involves informed choices, a balanced approach, and unwavering commitment.

So, take charge of your health today. Equip yourself with knowledge, make informed decisions, and stand tall—both metaphorically and literally—as you navigate the road to healthier, stronger bones. With a blend of social responsibility, individual freedom, and a dash of empirical evidence, you're not just managing osteoporosis; you're redefining what it means to live well.

Understanding the Absorption of Calcium and Magnesium Supplements

Understanding how calcium and magnesium supplements are absorbed can be pivotal in managing bone density and overall bone health, especially for adults who might be dealing with osteoporosis or other bone density issues. One key aspect to remember is that the absorption of these minerals doesn't occur in isolation but is influenced by various factors, including other vitamins and your general health.

Firstly, calcium absorption is significantly enhanced by vitamin D. You might already know that vitamin D plays a crucial role in calcium metabolism. Without adequate vitamin D, your body struggles to absorb the calcium you consume, making it less effective for maintaining your bone health. Here's what you can do for optimal effectiveness:

- Consider taking calcium and vitamin D supplements together. This combination helps ensure your body has what it needs to facilitate proper calcium absorption.

- Also, try incorporating vitamin D-rich foods into your diet, like fatty fish, egg yolks, and fortified dairy products, alongside your calcium supplements.

Spending time in sunlight can also boost your vitamin D levels, as your skin synthesizes this essential nutrient when exposed to UV rays.

Magnesium is another mineral that aids in calcium absorption and its utilization within the body. The interplay between these two minerals is quite fascinating and important. Magnesium actually helps regulate the transport of calcium across cell membranes, ensuring that calcium gets where it needs to go for bone formation and maintenance. For better bone health, balance your intake of magnesium and calcium.

- Make sure you're getting enough magnesium through supplements if necessary, or from food sources like leafy green vegetables, nuts, seeds, and whole grains.

- When choosing a supplement, look for one that includes both calcium and magnesium in appropriate ratios. This way, you support not just absorption but also the effective functioning of each mineral.

Age, vitamin deficiencies, and certain medications can affect how well your body absorbs these supplements. As we age, our bodies become less efficient at absorbing nutrients, which includes calcium and magnesium. Furthermore, some medications can interfere with the absorption process or increase the excretion of these minerals from our bodies. Similarly, deficiencies in other vitamins (like vitamin K2) can have cascading effects on how well calcium and magnesium are utilized.

If you're facing such absorption issues due to age, medications, or vitamin deficiencies, it's crucial to consult with a healthcare professional for personalized guidance. They can help you identify any potential gaps or interactions and adjust your supplement regimen accordingly. Personalized advice ensures that you're not just taking supplements, but you're taking them in a way that's most beneficial for your unique health circumstances.

Timing is another critical factor to consider. For many, taking calcium and magnesium supplements with meals can enhance their absorption and reduce the risk of side effects like gastrointestinal discomfort.

- Consuming these minerals alongside food stimulates stomach acid production, which helps break down the supplements more effectively.

- Additionally, spreading out the intake throughout the day rather than consuming them all at once can help improve absorption rates and maintain steady levels in your bloodstream.

It may sound like a lot to juggle, but understanding how calcium and magnesium supplements work can genuinely make a noticeable difference in your bone health. By integrating them thoughtfully into your routine, and paying attention to timing, complementary nutrients, and personal health factors, you can maximize their benefits.

In summary, the key takeaways should empower you to be more strategic with your supplement intake. Recognizing the role of vitamin D in calcium absorption, balancing magnesium intake, consulting healthcare professionals for tailored advice, and timing your supplements with meals are all actionable steps you can take. These measures ensure that you'll be supporting your bone density and overall bone health most effectively.

Remember, the goal here isn't just economic growth or convenience; it's about prioritizing human welfare, particularly your own health and well-being. Balancing your dietary intake and supplement regimen with an evidence-driven approach not only supports your bone health but also empowers you with the knowledge to make informed decisions. So next time you reach for your supplements, you'll know precisely why and how they fit into your broader health strategy.

Benefits of Combining Supplements for Optimal Bone Support

Exploring the benefits of combining supplements for optimal bone support can be transformative for your bone health. One of the most compelling areas of interest is how calcium, vitamin D, and magnesium can work together to provide a more robust defense against osteoporosis and other bone density issues.

Combining these three nutrients creates a synergistic effect. Calcium is, of course, vital as it is the primary component of bone tissue. However, calcium alone cannot do the job effectively. Vitamin D plays a crucial role in enhancing calcium absorption in the gut, ensuring that the calcium you consume is utilized efficiently. Magnesium complements both by helping to convert vitamin D into its active form and acting as a regulator for calcium transport. Together, they offer a powerful trio that supports better bone density.

To make the most out of these supplements, here are some steps you can take:

- **Start with a good quality calcium supplement:** Look for ones containing calcium citrate, which is generally absorbed better than other forms.

- **Ensure adequate vitamin D intake:** Depending on where you live and your exposure to sunlight, you might need anywhere from 600 to 2000 IU per day. Speak to your healthcare provider about appropriate levels.

- **Don't overlook magnesium:** You might want a supplement containing around 300-400 mg of magnesium citrate or glycinate for best results.

Incorporating other bone-supporting nutrients like vitamin K, zinc, and boron can further enhance this regimen. Vitamin K2 helps guide calcium to bones and prevents it from settling in arteries, which could cause arterial calcification. Zinc contributes to collagen production in the bone matrix, while boron aids in the efficient use of calcium and magnesium.

Here's how you can integrate these additional nutrients:

- **Vitamin K2:** Look for supplements containing MK-4 or MK-7 forms. Around 100 mcg daily is generally recommended for bone health.

- **Zinc:** A supplement providing about 10-15 mg of zinc citrate or gluconate should suffice.

- **Boron:** While less commonly known, a 3 mg daily dose of boron can do wonders for maximizing the effects of the other nutrients. In countries with boron rich soil, osteoporosis is nonexistent.

Creating a personalized supplement plan tailored to your specific needs and lifestyle is crucial. Consulting with a healthcare provider or a nutritionist can help you understand your unique requirements and design a regimen that's right for you. This step ensures that you're not taking redundant or excessive doses, which could be counterproductive or even harmful.

To get started on creating your plan:

- **Schedule an appointment with a healthcare provider or a nutritionist:** They will likely run some tests, such as blood work, to ascertain your current nutrient levels and bone density.

- **Discuss your lifestyle and dietary habits:** Based on your input, they'll craft a supplement plan tailored specifically to your needs.

- **Follow up periodically:** Keeping track of your progress can help fine-tune your regimen over time.

Regularly reviewing and adjusting your supplement intake is essential. Your needs may change based on various factors like age, health status, and lifestyle changes. For example, if you start a

new diet that includes more dairy or leafy greens, you might require less calcium supplementation. Alternatively, if you move to a region with little sunlight, you might need to up your vitamin D intake.

Here's how you can stay on top of your supplement routine:

- **Monitor your diet and lifestyle:** Keep a journal or use apps to track your nutrient intake and any lifestyle changes.

- **Stay in touch with healthcare professionals:** Regular check-ups can help catch any deficiencies early.

- **Adjust as necessary:** Don't hesitate to tweak your supplement intake based on new information or advice.

Synergistically combining various bone-supporting supplements can offer comprehensive benefits for bone density and overall bone health. Embracing a multi-nutrient approach rather than relying on a single supplement can provide a holistic solution to maintaining strong bones.

Engaging with evidence-based research and professional guidance empowers you to make informed decisions about your health.

Ultimately, your goal isn't just to pop a few pills and hope for the best; it's about integrating these supplements thoughtfully into your daily life. With the proper guidance and a willingness to adjust as you go, you'll be well on your way to optimal bone health.

Potential Risks of Excessive Supplementation

Excessive intake of calcium supplements can lead to several unintended consequences. While calcium is vital for maintaining strong bones, too much of it can result in kidney stones—a painful condition that many adults would rather avoid. Overloading on calcium can also disrupt the delicate balance of other essential minerals in your body. For instance, high levels of calcium can hinder the absorption of magnesium and zinc, both of which are crucial for overall health.

It's essential to adhere to recommended dosage guidelines when it comes to calcium supplementation. Here's what you can do to keep your calcium intake within safe limits: •   Consult with a healthcare provider for a tailored recommendation based on your specific needs.

- Follow the instructions on supplement labels diligently; they're usually designed to keep you within safe boundaries.

- Prioritize getting your calcium from food sources where possible, such as dairy products, leafy greens, and fortified foods.

Overconsumption of vitamin D supplements is another potential risk. Vitamin D works hand-in hand with calcium to strengthen bones, but taking it in excess can be harmful. High doses can lead to vitamin D toxicity, manifesting as symptoms like nausea, weakness, and elevated blood calcium levels. This imbalance can, in turn, lead to heart issues, bone pain, and even kidney problems.

To avoid these hazards, make sure to follow recommended dosages for vitamin D. Here's how:

- Check the daily intake guidelines provided by reputable health organizations.

- Combine your supplements thoughtfully. Sometimes, multivitamins contain vitamin D, so additional supplementation might not be necessary.

- Discuss your individual needs with a healthcare professional who can recommend an appropriate dosage based on your lifestyle and health status.

Regular monitoring of your calcium, magnesium, and vitamin D levels through blood tests is another crucial aspect of managing your bone health. These tests offer a snapshot of whether you're within the optimal range for maintaining strong and healthy bones. Blood tests can catch imbalances early, allowing for adjustments before any damage occurs.

Here's what you can do to monitor your levels effectively:

- Schedule regular check-ups with your healthcare provider to discuss your supplementation and diet.

- Request specific blood tests for calcium, magnesium, and vitamin D levels.

- Keep track of your test results over time to spot trends or changes.

But monitoring alone isn't enough. Professional guidance is indispensable when starting any new supplements. Your healthcare provider can offer personalized advice, ensuring that the supplements support your health goals without causing harm. If you experience any side effects or have concerns, it's important to bring them up immediately during consultations.

Here's how to seek professional guidance effectively:

- Make a list of all current medications and supplements you are taking, including dosages, to share with your healthcare provider.

- Jot down any symptoms or side effects you've noticed since starting a new supplement.

- Don't hesitate to ask questions about potential interactions with other supplements or medications.

Balancing your approach to supplementation is fundamental. Yes, supplements can play a significant role in bolstering bone density and overall health, but excessive intake can backfire, creating more problems than solutions. By being mindful of the dosages, regularly monitoring your nutrient levels, and seeking professional advice, you can reap the benefits while avoiding the pitfalls.

In summary, addressing potential risks of excessive supplementation requires a balanced approach. Too much calcium can lead to kidney stones and disrupt other minerals. Likewise, excessive vitamin D can bring about toxicity symptoms. Therefore, keeping tabs on your calcium, magnesium, and vitamin D levels through regular blood tests is essential. Finally, always seek professional guidance before adding new supplements to your regimen, and promptly address any concerns or side effects. This holistic approach ensures that you maximize the benefits of supplements while safeguarding your overall well-being.

Remember, the goal here is to enhance life quality, not complicate it. Adopting this conscientious, evidence-based strategy will help maintain strong bones and a healthier future. Taking control of your health through informed decisions will empower you, giving you both the freedom and the responsibility to manage your well-being effectively.

Balancing Supplements for Optimal Bone Health

In examining the role of supplements for bone health, we've discussed key elements like calcium, Vitamin D, magnesium, and collagen. Each plays a unique part in maintaining bone density and supporting overall skeletal strength. Our bones serve as a reservoir for these essential nutrients, and supplementing them ensures we mitigate deficits that could compromise our health.

Reflecting on our initial discussions, it becomes apparent that understanding and managing these supplements is crucial. Calcium is foundational, yet without sufficient Vitamin D, its efficiency plummets. Magnesium helps maintain equilibrium, converting Vitamin D to its active form, which then enhances calcium absorption. Collagen, often overlooked, contributes significantly to the structural integrity of our bones.

Currently, the emphasis lies on taking an informed and balanced approach to supplementation. Integrating these nutrients into your routine can offer substantial benefits. However, it's not merely about adding pills to your daily intake; it's about incorporating them thoughtfully and holistically. Balancing supplement use with dietary sources ensures that you're not overly reliant on one method, fostering better overall health.

Nevertheless, there are concerns worth noting. Excessive intake of any supplement can lead to issues such as kidney stones from too much calcium or toxicity from Vitamin D overuse. Ensuring safe dosages, regular monitoring, and professional guidance are critical steps to avoid these pitfalls.

The consequences of mismanaging supplements extend beyond individual health to public health at large. Widespread misuse of supplements can contribute to broader health crises, strain healthcare systems, and increase medical costs. Hence, responsible use based on empirical evidence and medical advice is paramount.

As you continue your journey towards better bone health, remember that knowledge and responsibility go hand in hand. By staying informed, making balanced choices, and seeking professional guidance, you empower yourself to navigate the complexities of osteoporosis management effectively. This strategy not only supports your physical well-being but also enhances your quality of life, setting a positive example for others navigating similar health challenges.

Chapter 6
Holistic Approaches to Osteoporosis

Living with osteoporosis often feels like walking a tightrope, balancing between managing symptoms and maintaining quality of life. The fear of fractures and the constant pain can make every movement feel like a calculated risk. Many people depend on conventional treatments such as medications and supplements, but there's a growing interest in holistic methods that can complement these traditional approaches. Holistic options aim not only to alleviate physical symptoms but also to enhance overall well-being, providing a more comprehensive treatment strategy for those affected by this bone condition.

Osteoporosis is characterized by weakened bones that are prone to fractures, often turning everyday activities into potential hazards. Conventional treatments, while effective to some extent, frequently fail to address the emotional and holistic aspects of living with this condition. For instance, medications might help slow down bone loss, yet they may not provide significant relief from chronic pain or improve emotional health. Additionally, the side effects of long-term medication use can be a concern for many patients. This gap in care has led individuals to seek out complementary therapies, hoping to find a more rounded approach to managing their condition. Acupuncture, aromatherapy, and mind-body practices have shown promise in filling these gaps, offering pain relief, reducing stress, and promoting better bone health.

In this chapter, we will explore various holistic approaches to managing osteoporosis naturally. We begin by examining the potential benefits of acupuncture, an ancient practice that stimulates specific points in the body to enhance bone health. Next, we delve into aromatherapy, highlighting how essential oils can be utilized for natural pain relief and emotional well-being. Finally, we discuss the role of mind-body practices such as yoga and mindfulness in improving flexibility, balance, and bone strength. By understanding these complementary therapies, readers can adopt a more integrative approach to their osteoporosis management, ultimately leading to a healthier and more fulfilling life.

Exploring the Benefits of Acupuncture

Acupuncture, though ancient in practice, has found its place in modern medicine as a promising complementary therapy for osteoporosis management. By stimulating specific points in the body associated with bone health, acupuncture encourages better circulation and aids in bone regeneration. This holistic approach can be transformative for individuals seeking to enhance their quality of life while managing osteoporosis.

When it comes to understanding how acupuncture works, it's essential to look at the mechanism behind it. Acupuncture involves the insertion of fine needles into predetermined points on the skin, known as acupoints. These acupoints correspond to various organs and systems in the body. For osteoporosis patients, targeted acupoints are believed to promote blood flow and nutrient supply to the bones, fostering an environment conducive to bone regeneration. Research suggests that this stimulation can lead to improved bone density over time.

Moreover, acupuncture is known to effectively reduce pain and inflammation—two significant challenges faced by those living with osteoporosis. Inflammation is a natural response to injury but becomes problematic when persistent. Chronic inflammation can exacerbate bone deterioration, making pain management a critical aspect of osteoporosis care. Acupuncture's anti-inflammatory

properties can help mitigate this issue, allowing patients to experience less discomfort and a higher quality of life.

For instance, studies have shown that regular acupuncture sessions can substantially lower levels of inflammatory markers in the body. Patients often report a decrease in pain intensity and frequency after consistent treatment, which in turn can reduce reliance on conventional pain medications. This not only alleviates physical symptoms but also addresses the emotional toll of chronic pain, contributing to overall well-being.

It's worth noting that, as beneficial as acupuncture can be, it must be administered by trained professionals to ensure both safety and effectiveness. Here are some guidelines to keep in mind:

- Ensure your acupuncturist is licensed and holds relevant certifications from reputable institutions. Verifying credentials helps protect you from potential harm due to improper technique or unsterilized equipment.

- Discuss your osteoporosis diagnosis and any other health conditions with your acupuncturist before starting treatment. Transparency allows them to tailor the sessions according to your specific needs and circumstances.

- Follow the recommended schedule for treatments, as consistency is key to achieving the desired outcomes. Skipping sessions can disrupt the therapeutic process and delay progress.

Incorporating acupuncture into a holistic treatment plan isn't about replacing conventional therapies but enhancing them. A balanced approach can yield the most comprehensive results. Traditional methods like prescription medications, weight-bearing exercises, and dietary changes remain vital. Yet, integrating acupuncture can add another layer of support, addressing aspects that might be overlooked by conventional means alone.

Patients who embrace such a multi-faceted approach often find themselves benefiting from the best of both worlds. For example, they might take medications that slow bone loss while practicing weight-bearing exercises to strengthen their skeletal system. Adding acupuncture into this mix can help manage pain and improve circulation, creating a more rounded and effective strategy for tackling osteoporosis.

Let's consider the case of Jane, a 65-year-old woman diagnosed with osteoporosis five years ago. Jane adhered to her doctor's recommendations, including calcium supplements and regular exercise. Despite these efforts, she still experienced significant back pain and stiffness. Upon her friend's suggestion, she decided to try acupuncture. After a few months of bi-weekly sessions, Jane noticed a remarkable reduction in her pain levels. Her mobility improved, and she felt more energetic during her daily activities. By working alongside her existing treatment regimen, acupuncture provided relief in areas previously unmanaged, showcasing its value in a comprehensive care plan.

Similarly, educational initiatives about acupuncture's role in osteoporosis management can empower patients. Understanding how and why acupuncture can benefit them allows individuals to make informed decisions about their health care. Healthcare providers should ideally include information sessions about alternative therapies, helping patients explore all viable options.

To summarize, acupuncture stands out as a valuable adjunct therapy for managing osteoporosis symptoms and enhancing overall bone health. Its ability to stimulate specific bodily points to promote better circulation and bone regeneration, coupled with its pain-relieving and antiinflammatory benefits, marks its significance in holistic osteoporosis care. Administered by trained professionals, acupuncture harmonizes with traditional treatments, offering a more nuanced approach to managing this condition. Therefore, for those open to alternative therapies, acupuncture may just be the complementary solution that bridges gaps left by conventional methods alone.

Using Aromatherapy for Natural Pain Relief

Aromatherapy, a practice deeply rooted in history and tradition, has emerged as a compelling holistic approach to managing the pain and anxiety often associated with osteoporosis. By harnessing the power of essential oils, individuals can not only alleviate physical discomfort but also enhance their emotional well-being. This is particularly significant given that osteoporosis doesn't just affect the bones; it impacts every facet of a person's life, from physical mobility to mental health.

Let's start by exploring how essential oils function within the context of aromatherapy. When we talk about using essential oils like lavender and peppermint, we're tapping into their natural analgesic properties. Lavender, for instance, is renowned for its calming effects, which can significantly reduce stress and anxiety levels—both common companions of chronic pain conditions such as osteoporosis. Imagine taking a deep breath with the gentle scent of lavender filling your lungs, providing immediate relaxation and a sense of peace. Peppermint, on the other hand, offers a cooling sensation and has been found to reduce muscle tension and pain, making it a versatile option for those dealing with bone-related discomfort.

For those wanting to incorporate these oils into their routine, here are some practical steps:

- Begin with high-quality, therapeutic-grade essential oils to ensure you receive the most benefit. • For topical application, dilute the essential oil with a carrier oil (like coconut or jojoba oil) before massaging it onto the affected area. A typical ratio is 2-3 drops of essential oil per teaspoon of carrier oil. This helps prevent any potential skin irritation.

- Inhale the aroma directly by adding a few drops of essential oil to a bowl of hot water or through an essential oil diffuser. This method allows the aromatic compounds to quickly reach the brain, promoting rapid stress relief and a mood uplift.

Incorporating aromatherapy into daily self-care routines can be straightforward and immensely rewarding. Picture this: after a long day, you create a peaceful ambiance by diffusing a mix of lavender and chamomile in your living space. As you settle down with a good book or perhaps meditate, the soothing scent envelops you, easing both body and mind. Regular use of these oils can build a calming ritual that integrates seamlessly into one's lifestyle, contributing to overall well-being and better managing osteoporosis symptoms.

Empirical evidence supporting the efficacy of aromatherapy adds weight to its consideration as a viable complementary therapy. Studies have shown that consistent use of certain essential oils can lead to measurable reductions in pain levels and improvements in mood. This isn't just anecdotal; research data provides a firm foundation for these claims, giving us a reason to be optimistic about integrating aromatherapy into broader osteoporosis management plans.

There's no denying that living with osteoporosis poses unique challenges, particularly when it comes to maintaining quality of life. Beyond pharmaceutical interventions, it's crucial to consider complementary therapies that address both the physical and emotional dimensions of this condition. Aromatherapy stands out because it is non-invasive, easy to implement, and can be tailored to individual preferences and needs.

When looking at the broader picture, it's clear that holistic methods like aromatherapy represent a marriage between empirical evidence and personal empowerment. They offer a way for individuals to take control of their own health and well-being within the framework of scientifically backed practices. This balance between self-care and supported medical approaches creates a more comprehensive strategy for tackling osteoporosis.

One point that deserves emphasis is the importance of integrating aromatherapy with conventional treatments under professional guidance. It's essential to consult healthcare providers before starting any new therapy, even something as seemingly benign as essential oils. By doing so, you ensure that all aspects of your care are harmonized and that there are no unintended interactions with prescribed medications or other treatments.

A key takeaway here is the immense value in viewing health through a multifaceted lens. Pain and discomfort are not merely physical—they affect our mental state, our social interactions, and ultimately, our overall quality of life. Embracing aromatherapy as part of a holistic approach underscores the commitment to treating the whole person rather than just a set of symptoms.

Let's delve a bit deeper into specific essential oils and their uses. Besides lavender and peppermint, oils like eucalyptus and frankincense also hold promise. Eucalyptus oil, known for its anti-inflammatory properties, can help ease joint and muscle pain. Similarly, frankincense has been used for centuries in traditional medicine for its ability to promote cellular health and reduce inflammation. Incorporating these oils into regular massage or inhalation routines can offer additional layers of pain relief and emotional support.

To sum up, aromatherapy provides a compelling, evidence-backed method to enhance the lives of those dealing with osteoporosis. It aligns the reduction of physical pain with the promotion of emotional wellness, offering a balanced approach that respects both the scientific and personal aspects of health management. By carefully selecting and using essential oils, people can find relief and comfort in ways that complement their existing treatment regimens.

Imagine creating a sanctuary in your own home—an environment where the scents of nature contribute to healing and tranquility. Through such holistic practices, we make strides not just in managing the symptoms of osteoporosis but in enriching the overall human experience. And that, fundamentally, is what good healthcare should strive to achieve: a harmonious blend of science, compassion, and personal empowerment.

Mind-Body Practices for Stress Reduction

Exploring mind-body practices for stress reduction and overall well-being in individuals with osteoporosis holds significant promise. It's fascinating how interconnected our physical health is with our mental and emotional states. When dealing with conditions like osteoporosis, managing stress effectively can have a profound impact on bone health.

Mind-Body Techniques for Lowering Stress Hormones

Stress hormones such as cortisol can negatively affect bone density, making it crucial to manage stress levels. Engaging in mind-body techniques like meditation and deep breathing can be incredibly beneficial. These practices are designed to lower the body's stress response, thereby minimizing the release of harmful stress hormones.

To incorporate these techniques:

- Start with finding a quiet space where you won't be disturbed.

- Sit or lie down comfortably, closing your eyes to focus inward.

- Begin by taking slow, deep breaths, inhaling through your nose and exhaling through your mouth.

- Concentrate on each breath, allowing your thoughts to pass without judgment.

- Allocate about 10-15 minutes per session initially and gradually extend the time as you become more comfortable.

By consciously practicing these simple steps, you begin to train your body to respond to stress more calmly. Over time, this can significantly contribute to maintaining better bone health.

Regular Practice of Mindfulness for Improved Sleep and Reduced Anxiety

Mindfulness is another powerful tool that can improve sleep quality, reduce anxiety, and enhance the body's natural healing processes. When we talk about mindfulness, we're essentially talking about being present in the moment, fully aware, and engaged.

Here are practical steps to get started:

- Set aside dedicated time each day, preferably at the same hour, to practice mindfulness.

- Use a comfortable chair or cushion. Keep your back straight but not rigid, to remain alert yet relaxed.

- Focus your attention on your breathing or on bodily sensations, bringing your mind back gently whenever it wanders.

Over time, consistent practice can lead to improved sleep patterns and reduced anxiety levels, both of which are beneficial for anyone managing osteoporosis. The connection between good sleep and bone health shouldn't be underestimated; while we sleep, our body undergoes critical repair and rebuilding processes, including those involved in maintaining bone density.

Promoting Relaxation and Mental Clarity through Mind-Body Practices

Relaxation and mental clarity are attainable outcomes through regular engagement in mind-body practices, crucial for managing the complexities of osteoporosis. Methods like progressive muscle relaxation, guided imagery, and yoga provide not only physical benefits but also cultivate a sense of inner calm and mental sharpness.

For example, progressive muscle relaxation involves:

- Gradually tensing and then relaxing different muscle groups in the body.

- Starting from your toes and moving upwards to your face.

- Holding the tension for a few seconds before releasing it completely.

By systematically working through your muscle groups, you can ease physical tension, which often accumulates due to stress. This practice enhances relaxation and can indirectly support bone health by lowering overall stress levels.

Integrating Mind-Body Exercises into Daily Routines

Integrating these mind-body exercises into your daily routine can support emotional resilience and optimize bone health outcomes. It's one thing to understand the benefits theoretically, but how do you practically fit these techniques into a busy life?

Consider these suggestions:

- Incorporate short sessions of deep breathing or meditation into your morning routine.

- Use mid-day breaks for quick mindfulness exercises, even if it's just a couple of minutes of focused breathing.

- Wind down in the evening with progressive muscle relaxation or gentle yoga stretches to prepare for a restful night's sleep.

Making these practices part of your daily schedule ensures they become habitual, fostering longterm benefits for both mental and physical health.

Holistic Strategies for Managing Osteoporosis

In summary, mind-body practices offer holistic strategies to manage stress, enhance emotional well-being, and support bone health in individuals with osteoporosis. While medications and physical therapies play crucial roles in treating this condition, incorporating holistic methods can provide additional layers of support.

The beauty of these techniques lies in their simplicity and accessibility. You don't need any special equipment, just a bit of time, commitment, and the willingness to explore how deeply interconnected your mind and body truly are. By acknowledging and nurturing this connection, you empower yourself toward better overall health and well-being.

Engaging in debates and discussions about the effectiveness of these methods reveals a variety of perspectives. Yet, the empirical evidence supporting the positive impacts of mind-body practices on stress and overall health continues to grow. Therefore, embracing these methods can serve as a complementary approach to your existing treatment plan, ensuring a balanced pathway to managing osteoporosis.

Ultimately, the goal is to foster an environment of well-being where stress is managed effectively, and emotional resilience is nurtured, leading to optimal bone health outcomes.

Here's to integrating mindfulness, meditation, and relaxation into your daily life, paving the way for healthier bones and a more centered mind.

Yoga for Flexibility, Balance, and Bone Strength

When it comes to managing osteoporosis, many people often think of medications and dietary supplements as their primary tools. However, holistic methods and alternative therapies can play a crucial role in addressing this condition naturally. One such holistic method is yoga, which offers numerous benefits for those dealing with osteoporosis. Engaging in yoga not only helps improve flexibility and balance but also strengthens bones, making it an excellent complementary approach to traditional osteoporosis treatment plans.

Yoga poses and stretches can help increase bone density, muscle strength, and joint flexibility. Incorporating specific yoga exercises into your daily routine can target key areas affected by osteoporosis. For example, the Tree Pose, where you stand on one leg and bring the opposite foot to rest on your inner thigh, helps foster both balance and strength in your leg and core muscles. Additionally, poses like the Warrior series engage multiple muscle groups simultaneously, promoting increased bone density over time.

In order to maximize these benefits:

- Begin with basic yoga poses and gradually progress to more advanced ones as your strength and flexibility improve.

- Utilize props like yoga blocks and straps to support yourself in poses, reducing the risk of strain or injury.

- Focus on maintaining proper alignment and posture in each pose to ensure maximum effectiveness and safety.

Weight-bearing yoga exercises stimulate bone-building cells, promoting skeletal health and reducing fracture risk. Essentially, when we perform certain yoga poses that require our body to work against gravity, it sends signals to our bones, encouraging them to become stronger and denser. Poses such as Downward-Facing Dog and Plank engage the arms, legs, and core, creating a natural resistance that enhances bone strength. These poses mimic weight-bearing activities that are often recommended for osteoporosis management.

To effectively incorporate weight-bearing yoga exercises:

- Start with short sessions, around 10-15 minutes, and gradually extend the duration as you become more comfortable and confident.

- Pay attention to your body's feedback; if a pose causes discomfort or pain, modify it or choose a different one.

- Practice consistently, aiming for at least three times a week to reap the long-term benefits for bone health.

Yoga practice enhances body awareness, improves posture, and boosts overall physical function in individuals with osteoporosis. When practicing yoga, there's a strong emphasis on connecting mind and body through breath control and mindful movement. This heightened body awareness contributes to better posture, which is particularly important for individuals with osteoporosis who may suffer from spine curvature or other postural issues. Enhanced posture not only reduces the likelihood of falls but also supports overall spinal health, minimizing the risk of fractures.

To enhance body awareness and improve posture through yoga:

- Focus on breathing techniques that synchronize with your movements, fostering a deeper connection between mind and body.

- Include poses that elongate the spine and open up the chest, such as Cobra Pose and CatCow stretches.

- Partner with a qualified yoga instructor who understands the needs of individuals with osteoporosis and can provide personalized guidance.

Regular participation in yoga classes or home practice can complement osteoporosis treatment plans and contribute to a holistic approach to bone health. By integrating yoga into your routine, you create an environment where physical activity becomes more than just exercise—it becomes a way of enhancing your overall well-being. Whether you choose to join a local yoga class or follow online sessions from the comfort of your home, consistency is key. Not only does regular yoga practice strengthen your bones, but it also relieves stress, promotes relaxation, and enhances mental clarity—all integral parts of managing osteoporosis holistically.

To maintain a consistent yoga practice:

- Schedule specific times for yoga sessions throughout the week, treating them as nonnegotiable appointments with yourself.

- Create a dedicated space in your home where you can practice without distractions, even if it's just a small corner with a yoga mat.

- Incorporate both variety and repetition in your routines to keep them engaging while reinforcing familiar poses.

This brings us to the holistic power of yoga. It offers a gentle yet effective way to enhance bone strength, flexibility, and overall well-being for individuals managing osteoporosis. Unlike highimpact exercises, yoga is unlikely to place undue stress on weakened bones, making it a safe option for many. The slow, deliberate movements allow for control and precision, reducing the chances of injury. Furthermore, yoga's emphasis on harmony between mind and body ensures that individuals do not just work on their physical state but also achieve a sense of mental peace and emotional balance, ultimately contributing to a comprehensive approach to health.

Do note that while yoga is beneficial, it is essential to consult healthcare providers before beginning any new exercise regimen, especially for those with osteoporosis. This ensures that the selected yoga practices align well with individual health conditions and treatment plans. They can offer tailored advice and might even recommend specific types of yoga or instructors trained to work with osteoporosis patients.

In conclusion, weaving yoga into your lifestyle can significantly bolster your fight against osteoporosis. It works on multiple fronts: increasing bone density, improving muscle strength, enhancing flexibility, promoting body awareness, and supporting mental and emotional wellbeing. The key lies in starting slowly, remaining consistent, and seeking professional guidance to tailor your practice to your unique needs. With its multifaceted benefits, yoga stands out as a remarkable alternative therapy that complements traditional treatments, offering a holistic path to managing osteoporosis.

Integrating Holistic Therapies for Optimal Bone Health

Throughout this chapter, we've delved into various holistic methods and alternative therapies for managing osteoporosis naturally. From the ancient practice of acupuncture to the aromatic wonders of essential oils and the mindful movements of yoga, each approach offers unique benefits that complement traditional osteoporosis treatments. These methods do not replace conventional practices but rather enhance them, providing a more rounded strategy to improving bone health and overall well-being.

Acupuncture has shown promise in stimulating specific points in the body to promote better circulation and bone regeneration. It can significantly reduce pain and inflammation, allowing individuals to manage their symptoms more effectively. Similarly, aromatherapy uses the power of essential oils to alleviate physical discomfort and boost emotional wellness, making it a valuable tool in the holistic management of osteoporosis. Essential oils like lavender and peppermint offer natural analgesic properties that can ease muscle tension and create a calming environment, which is crucial for managing chronic conditions.

We've seen how incorporating mind-body practices such as meditation and mindfulness can lower stress levels and improve sleep quality. Stress hormones negatively impact bone density, and these techniques offer a way to mitigate those effects. By fostering relaxation and mental clarity, mind-body practices support both emotional resilience and bone health. Additionally, yoga stands out as an exercise that enhances flexibility, balance, and bone strength. Its weightbearing poses stimulate bone-building cells, promoting skeletal health without undue stress on the bones.

However, it's essential to approach these therapies with caution and professional guidance. Consulting healthcare providers ensures that these methods align well with individual health conditions and existing treatment plans. This is particularly important for people with severe osteoporosis or other underlying health issues.

Embracing these holistic approaches has broader implications. They represent a shift toward treating the whole person rather than just addressing specific symptoms. This comprehensive view acknowledges that physical health is deeply intertwined with mental and emotional states. The integration of these therapies into one's lifestyle can lead to enhanced quality of life and overall well-being.

As we continue to explore alternative and complementary therapies, it's vital to keep an open mind and consider all viable options. The journey towards better bone health isn't about choosing one path over another but finding a balanced approach that works best for the individual. Through this, we move closer to a holistic understanding of health—one that respects the complex interplay between mind, body, and spirit. With every step taken in this direction, we're not just managing osteoporosis; we're enriching the human experience.

Chapter 7
Bone Health Across the Lifespan

Bones are the silent guardians of our bodies, providing structure, protection, and support for daily activities. Yet, often we give little thought to their health until a problem arises. Just as a building must be constructed on a solid foundation to stand the test of time, so too must our bones be strong from the start to support us throughout our lives. This chapter delves into the journey of bone health across various stages of life, highlighting the importance of nurturing our skeletal system through every phase of development and aging.

The issue of bone health becomes apparent when considering the prevalence of conditions like osteoporosis, a disease characterized by brittle and fragile bones that affects millions worldwide. In youth, failing to achieve peak bone mass can set the stage for future problems. For example, inadequate calcium intake or lack of physical activity during childhood can lead to weaker bones, making them more susceptible to fractures. As individuals age, bone density naturally begins to decrease, sometimes leading to serious complications if not properly managed. Adults must remain vigilant about their lifestyle choices, including nutrition and exercise, to mitigate the effects of aging on their bone health.

This chapter will provide insights into how bone health can be promoted at every life stage. We'll explore practical strategies for children and adolescents to build strong bones early on, such as consuming calcium-rich foods and participating in weight-bearing activities. Moving into adulthood, the focus shifts to maintaining bone density through balanced diets rich in calcium and vitamin D, regular exercise, and avoiding harmful habits like smoking and excessive drinking. By understanding and implementing these strategies, readers can take proactive steps to ensure their bones remain strong and resilient throughout their lives.

Promoting Bone Health in Youth

Understanding bone development during childhood and adolescence is pivotal for long term bone health. During these formative years, the body builds peak bone mass, which serves as a critical defense against osteoporosis in later life. The foundation of strong bones is laid early on, much like the foundation of a house. If that base is solid, it ensures resilience and durability throughout life.

One of the fundamental steps in nurturing this base is encouraging sufficient calcium intake during growth years. Calcium is the building block of our bones. Without it, bones can become brittle and more prone to fractures. So, how do we ensure kids get enough calcium? Here are some practical guidelines:

- **Incorporate Dairy Products:** Foods such as milk, cheese, and yogurt are rich in calcium.

- **Explore Fortified Foods:** Many products like orange juice and cereals are fortified with calcium.

- **Diverse Diet:** Include leafy greens like kale and broccoli, which also provide substantial amounts of calcium.

- **Calcium Supplements:** If dietary sources are insufficient, consider consulting a healthcare provider about supplements.

While milk can be a good source of calcium, too much can have the opposite effect. Women that drink three or more glasses of milk a day increase the chance of hip fractures. In tandem with calcium intake, engaging in weight-bearing activities during youth can significantly enhance bone strength and durability. Activities such as running and jumping apply pressure to the bones, stimulating them to become denser and stronger. When children engage in regular physical activity, they subject their bones to varied stresses, prompting bones to adapt and grow more resiliently. To encourage this:

- **Organize Playdates And Physical Activities:** This could include games of tag, hopscotch, or sports like soccer and basketball.

- **Encourage Participation in Sports:** Enroll children in activities like gymnastics, tennis, or track and field.

- **Promote Active Play:** Simple activities like jumping rope or playing on playground equipment can be highly beneficial.

Moreover, educating parents on the importance of promoting bone health habits in their children lays the groundwork for lifelong skeletal wellness. Parents play an essential role in shaping their children's habits and ensuring they get the right nutrients and exercise. By adopting healthy practices early, children can carry these good habits into adulthood. Here's what parents can do:

- **Lead By Example:** Children often emulate their parents. When parents maintain a diet rich in calcium and engage in regular physical activities, children are likely to follow suit. Limit your sugar intake, especially soda like drinks. Studies have shown they have a detrimental effect on our bones due to the phosphoric acid in the drinks.

- **Make Nutrition Fun:** Use creative ways to include calcium-rich foods in meals, such as preparing smoothies with yogurt and fruits or making homemade pizzas with plenty of cheese and veggie toppings.

- **Allocate Time for Family Exercises:** Plan regular family outings that involve physical activities, such as hiking, biking, or even dancing at home.

During the growth period, the skeleton is constantly undergoing changes through bone modeling and remodeling, which is a process of optimizing bone strength. Bone strength is especially "tested" during growth and aging periods, as the incidence of fractures is higher in these stages of life (Baptista et al., 2022). Obesity seems to be a risk factor for bone fractures despite a greater mechanical load associated with overweight and obesity. Bone tissue is negatively influenced by the inflammatory state caused by cytokines released from adipose tissue (Baptista et al., 2022).

Educating both children and adolescents about the importance of maintaining a healthy weight is equally crucial. Teaching them balanced eating habits and the benefits of regular exercise can prevent obesity-related issues and promote better bone health. Schools can also be a significant ally in this education, incorporating nutrition and physical education into their curricula.

The concept of peak bone mass—the maximum amount of bone mass reached between the second and third decade of life—is critical for bone strength. It's akin to reaching the pinnacle of a hill; how high you get determines how far you can see and how sturdy you stand against gusts of wind. Factors influencing peak bone mass include nutritional intake, hormonal balance, and physical activity levels. Therefore, monitoring and supporting these factors from an early age can have profound effects.

For instance, adequate vitamin D levels are essential for calcium absorption and bone health. Encouraging safe sun exposure and considering food sources like fatty fish, egg yolks, and fortified foods can help maintain optimal vitamin D levels. In cases where dietary intake and sunlight exposure are insufficient, supplements might be necessary under medical advice.

As children transition into adolescence, their hormonal changes significantly impact bone development. Estrogen, particularly in girls, plays a crucial role in bone metabolism. Ensuring that adolescent girls receive appropriate guidance on maintaining a balanced diet and engaging in physical activities is vital for achieving peak bone mass.

It's also essential to recognize that genetics play a notable role in determining bone density and overall skeletal health. While we can't change genetic predispositions, being aware of familial patterns can prompt proactive measures. Families with histories of osteoporosis should be particularly vigilant about bone health strategies.

Creating a supportive environment for bone health involves multiple stakeholders— parents, schools, healthcare providers, and community programs. It's a collaborative effort to instill habits that favor long-term skeletal wellness. For instance, healthcare providers can regularly check children's bone density when necessary and offer personalized advice based on individual needs.

Community programs focusing on children's sports and fitness can be instrumental in providing accessible platforms for weight-bearing activities. Local governments and organizations can establish affordable sports leagues or after-school programs that encourage active lifestyles, ensuring that all children, regardless of socioeconomic status, have opportunities to strengthen their bones.

In summary, understanding bone development during childhood and adolescence is crucial for long-term bone health. Encouraging a diet rich in calcium and engaging children in regular, weight-bearing physical activities can significantly influence their bone density and strength. Educating parents and creating supportive environments are essential steps in fostering habits that will sustain lifelong skeletal wellness. By taking evidence-driven actions and collaborating across various sectors, we can ensure that our future generations stand strong on the firm foundation of robust bone health.

Maintaining Strong Bones Through Adulthood

In adulthood, maintaining a balanced diet rich in calcium and vitamin D supports bone health and minimizes bone loss. The importance of these nutrients cannot be overstated. Calcium is vital for building and maintaining strong bones, while vitamin D helps your body absorb calcium more efficiently. Without adequate levels of these nutrients, bones can become brittle and weak over time, increasing the risk of osteoporosis and fractures.

To ensure you're getting enough calcium and vitamin D, consider incorporating dairy products like milk, cheese, and yogurt into your daily diet. If you're lactose intolerant or vegan, look towards leafy green vegetables, almonds, and fortified foods such as cereals and soy products. Additionally, spending short periods outside in the sun can help your body produce vitamin D naturally. However, you may also need supplements to reach the recommended daily intake of 1,200 mg of calcium and 600-800 IUs of vitamin D, especially as you age (Mayo Clinic, 2022).

Regular physical activity, including weight-bearing exercises and strength training, helps preserve bone density in adulthood. Exercise is crucial because it stimulates bone formation and slows down bone loss. Weight-bearing exercises, such as walking, jogging, dancing, and stair climbing, put stress on your bones in a healthy way, encouraging them to rebuild and remain strong. Similarly, resistance training exercises like lifting weights, using resistance bands, or body-weight workouts such as push-ups and squats, significantly contribute to bone health by strengthening the muscles surrounding the bones, which adds an extra layer of protection against fractures (Branch, 2023).

Here is what you can do in order to achieve this goal:

- Incorporate at least 150 minutes of moderate-intensity exercise into your weekly routine.

- Combine this with muscle-strengthening activities at least twice a week.

- Try to mix different types of physical activities to engage various muscle groups and keep workouts interesting.

- Always consult a healthcare provider before starting any new exercise program, especially if you have existing health issues.

Avoiding smoking and excessive alcohol consumption can reduce the risk of bone-related issues in adulthood. Smoking has been shown to impede the body's ability to absorb calcium, weakening bone structure over time. Similarly, excessive alcohol intake interferes with the balance of calcium in the body, leading to bone loss and increased fracture risk. For optimal bone health, it's advisable to quit smoking altogether and limit alcohol intake to moderate levels—defined as up to one drink per day for women and up to two drinks per day for men (Bone Health Basics - OrthoInfo - AAOS, n.d.).

Educating adults on the importance of regular bone density screenings to monitor bone health status is also vital. These screenings are essential for early detection of bone loss conditions, such as osteoporosis, that may not exhibit noticeable symptoms until significant damage has already occurred. Regular screenings allow healthcare providers to track changes in bone density over time and recommend appropriate interventions to prevent further bone loss.

To stay proactive about monitoring your bone health:

- Schedule regular bone density tests, especially if you are over 50 or have risk factors for osteoporosis.

- Discuss the results with your healthcare provider to understand your bone health status.

- Based on your screening results, follow any recommendations your doctor provides, which may include lifestyle changes or medications.

Understanding individual risk factors for poor bone health can further empower you to take charge of your well-being. Genetic factors play a significant role in determining bone density, but lifestyle choices such as diet, exercise, and avoiding harmful substances can mitigate some of these risks. For those with a family history of osteoporosis or related conditions, being extra vigilant about bone health practices is even more crucial.

Maintaining bone health is indeed a multi-faceted approach that combines nutrition, exercise, lifestyle decisions, and medical oversight. Balancing economic growth with human welfare means ensuring that accessible and affordable solutions for maintaining bone health are available to everyone. Individual freedom in making lifestyle choices should be complemented by social responsibility, such as public health campaigns promoting bone health awareness and government policies that support affordable healthcare services, including bone density screenings and preventive measures against osteoporosis.

The synergy between personal responsibility and societal support forms the backbone of improved public health outcomes. When individuals make informed decisions based on empirical evidence and recommended guidelines, and when governments and corporations provide the necessary support structures, the collective move towards better bone health becomes achievable. This balanced approach reflects my belief in the power of data-driven policy that respects both personal freedom and the necessity of a safety net for those who face hard times.

For a society to thrive, its members must have the information and resources they need to maintain their health. By placing human welfare above all, we create an environment where economic growth serves the people, ensuring that advancements reach every individual, particularly in the realm of health. Bone health, though a single aspect of overall wellbeing, encapsulates the crucial intersection of personal action and social support—a model that can and should extend across all areas of health care, housing, education, and beyond.

In conclusion, taking steps to maintain strong bones throughout adulthood involves a combination of a nutrient-rich diet, consistent physical activity, avoiding harmful habits, and staying informed through regular health screenings. Each of these elements plays an integral role in supporting bone health, ultimately contributing to a healthier, more resilient population. With evidence-based strategies and a collaborative approach between individuals, healthcare providers, and policymakers, we can work towards a future where robust bone health is a standard part of life, enhancing overall quality and longevity.

Lifelong Bone Health: A Continuous Effort

Understanding the significance of bone health from a young age sets the stage for strong bones throughout life. We've discussed how childhood and adolescence are critical periods for building peak bone mass, which can protect against osteoporosis later. Fundamental to this is ensuring adequate calcium intake and vitamin D levels, as well as engaging in weight-bearing activities that encourage bone strength.

Reflecting on the analogy introduced earlier, the foundation of a house must be solid to ensure resilience and durability over time. This metaphor underscores our position: prioritizing bone health early can lead to stronger, more resilient bones in adulthood. Parents, educators, and healthcare providers play pivotal roles in fostering these habits. Kids learn from their environments; therefore, creating an atmosphere that emphasizes healthy eating and regular physical activity is essential.

However, not everyone may find it easy to maintain these practices consistently. Barriers such as socioeconomic factors, lack of access to nutritious foods, or insufficient opportunities for physical activity can hinder efforts to build a solid bone health foundation. Consequently, communities and policymakers must work together to provide resources and support systems that cater to all children, regardless of their background. Without these interventions, the risk of widespread bone health issues looms large, potentially leading to increased healthcare costs and reduced quality of life in the future.

On a broader scale, addressing bone health from an early age influences public health positively. Stronger bones contribute to fewer fractures, less disability, and lower healthcare expenses in the long term. These benefits extend beyond the individual, enhancing societal well-being and economic stability.

As we conclude, consider the steps each of us can take—whether as parents, educators, or community members—to lay a firm foundation for our children's bone health. The investments made today in promoting healthy habits can yield immeasurable benefits for generations to come. Encouraging simple yet effective strategies for bone health now can help ensure a future where robust, healthy bones are the norm, paving the way for a healthier society overall.

References

National Institute of Arthritis and Musculoskeletal and Skin Diseases. (2023). *Exercise for Your Bone Health*. Retrieved from https://www.niams.nih.gov/health-topics/exercise-yourbone-health

Mayo Clinic. (2022). *How to keep your bones healthy*. Retrieved from https://www.mayoclinic.org/healthy-lifestyle/adult-health/in-depth/bone-health/art20045060

American Academy of Orthopaedic Surgeons. (n.d.). *Bone Health Basics - OrthoInfo - AAOS*. Retreived from https://www.orthoinfo.org/en/staying-healthy/bone-health-basics/

Baronio, F., & Baptista, F. (2022). *Editorial: Bone health and development in children and adolescents. Frontiers in Endocrinology*, 13(10), 1101403. https://doi.org/10.3389/fendo.2022.1101403

Levine, M. A. (2012). *Assessing bone health in children and adolescents. Indian Journal of Endocrinology and Metabolism*, 16(Suppl 2), S205. https://doi.org/10.4103/22308210.104040

Chapter 8

Mind-Body Connection in Bone Health

Bone health is far more than just the strength of our skeletal system; it's intricately connected to the well-being of our mind. The concept of the mind-body connection is gaining traction in both scientific and medical communities. This chapter delves into how mental well-being can significantly impact bone health, especially in the context of osteoporosis management. By understanding this relationship, individuals can adopt a holistic approach to maintaining and enhancing their bone density through not only physical but also psychological interventions.

Chronic stress is an insidious adversary that affects many facets of our health, including bone density. When the body is under sustained stress, it produces elevated levels of cortisol—a hormone known for its detrimental effects on bone-building cells. Over time, this hormonal imbalance can accelerate bone deterioration, exacerbating conditions like osteoporosis. For example, someone constantly dealing with high-stress situations might unknowingly be undermining their skeletal strength due to prolonged cortisol exposure. It's a stark reminder that mental health isn't just about emotional balance but also about safeguarding vital aspects of our physical health.

In this chapter, we will explore various mind-body techniques designed to mitigate the harmful effects of chronic stress on bone health. From mindfulness practices like meditation and deepbreathing exercises to stress management strategies through hobbies and yoga, the chapter offers actionable advice. We will also discuss the importance of professional help for those struggling to manage stress independently. By integrating these techniques into daily routines, individuals can better manage stress hormone levels and subsequently protect their bones from deterioration, fostering a holistic approach to managing osteoporosis.

Understanding the Role of Stress in Bone Density Loss

Chronic stress often sneaks up on us, silently impacting our lives in numerous ways. One of its lesser-known effects is on bone density. When we experience chronic stress, our bodies increase the production of cortisol, a hormone that, when consistently elevated, can lead to bone loss (Chin et al., 2021). Over time, high cortisol levels can interfere with bone-building cells and enhance the activity of bone-resorbing cells, which naturally leads to decreased bone density.

So, how do we combat this stress-induced bone deterioration? One of the most effective approaches is through mind-body techniques. Mind-body practices like meditation and deep breathing exercises are more than just relaxation strategies—they actively reduce stress hormones and promote overall bone health.

Here is what you can do in order to achieve the goal:

- Find a quiet place where you can sit or lie down comfortably.

- Close your eyes and take several deep breaths, focusing on inhaling deeply and exhaling slowly.

- Practice this for about 10-15 minutes daily, gradually increasing the duration as you get more comfortable.

By incorporating these simple practices into your daily routine, you can help lower cortisol levels, thereby protecting your bones from potential harm.

Expanding upon these practices, engaging in regular stress management activities can also make a considerable difference. Hobbies, yoga, and spending time in nature are wonderful options to consider for managing stress effectively. Each of these activities contributes not only to mental well-being but also promotes physical health.

To manage stress through hobbies and activities:

- Identify activities you enjoy and find fulfilling, whether it's painting, gardening, or playing an instrument.

- Make time for these activities regularly, aiming for at least once or twice a week.

- Consider joining groups or communities that share your interests; social interaction can be incredibly beneficial for reducing stress.

Spending time in nature has been proven to have calming effects. Nature encourages us to slow down, breathe, and appreciate the world around us, which can significantly reduce stress levels.

To integrate nature into your life:

- Plan regular walks in parks, forests, or along beaches. Aim for at least 30 minutes per session.

- If possible, bring elements of nature into your home, such as plants or natural light.

- Engage in outdoor activities like hiking or bird-watching to stay active while enjoying the benefits of nature.

Managing life's stressors isn't always something we can handle alone. Seeking professional help or therapy can be a crucial step in addressing underlying issues affecting your stress levels and, consequently, your bone health. Therapists can offer tools and strategies tailored to your specific situation, providing you with a structured approach to deal with stress.

Here is what you can do to seek professional help:

- Reach out to a licensed therapist or counselor who specializes in stress management or cognitive-behavioral therapy.

- Be open to trying different types of therapy, such as individual counseling, group therapy, or even teletherapy.

- Engage actively in the therapeutic process, setting goals and working towards them with your therapist's guidance.

In summation, understanding the impact of stress on bone density and learning how to manage it effectively is crucial for maintaining both bone density and overall well-being. By leveraging mind-body techniques, engaging in stress-reducing activities, and seeking professional help when needed, we can protect our bones and enhance our quality of life. Managing stress is not just about preserving bone health; it's about fostering a holistic sense of wellness that benefits every aspect of our lives.

So, let's take proactive steps today. Incorporate meditation and deep breathing into your routine, indulge in hobbies, practice yoga, spend more time in nature, and don't hesitate to seek professional advice. Your bones—and your whole self—will thank you.

Introducing Mindfulness Practices for Overall Health

When we talk about mental well-being and bone health, the relationship may not seem immediately obvious. However, scientific research continues to unveil how the two are deeply interconnected. By enhancing our mental clarity and focus, mindfulness practices can positively influence our overall bone density, proving to be a powerful tool in managing osteoporosis.

Mindfulness techniques can help individuals become more aware of their mental and emotional states, leading to reduced stress and improved bone health. The act of consistently bringing one's attention to the present moment can significantly reduce chronic stress—a known inhibitor of bone density. Stress triggers the release of cortisol, a hormone that can weaken bones over time.

When mindful practices such as meditation or deep-breathing exercises are regularly incorporated into one's daily routine, they can buffer against these harmful hormonal impacts.

Moving on to mindfulness meditation specifically, this practice has been shown to enhance mental clarity and focus. Enhanced mental clarity means better decision-making, especially concerning lifestyle choices that affect bone health. For instance, being present and focused allows one to adhere more strictly to prescribed medications or recommended dietary adjustments essential for managing osteoporosis. To incorporate mindfulness meditation effectively into your daily life:

- Find a quiet space where you won't be disturbed.

- Sit comfortably with your back straight yet relaxed.

- Close your eyes and start by focusing on your breath, noticing how it moves in and out.

- When thoughts intrude, gently guide your focus back to your breathing.

- Aim to practice for at least 10 minutes daily, gradually increasing the duration as you get more comfortable.

Incorporating mindfulness into daily routines also proves beneficial. Consider mindful eating and mindful movement. Mindful eating involves savoring each bite, paying close attention to the food's taste, texture, and nutritional benefits, thereby fostering healthier eating habits that provide vital nutrients for bone health. Similarly, mindful movement practices like yoga or Tai Chi not only build physical strength and balance but also promote bone density improvement (Global Health NOW, 2017; Lu et al., 2020). These practices encourage gentle yet effective weightbearing activities, which are crucial for maintaining bone mass.

To integrate these practices into daily life, here are some guidelines:

- During meals, take a moment to appreciate the food before you begin eating. Chew slowly and relish each flavor.

- Practice yoga or Tai Chi for at least 20 minutes three times a week. Focus on movements that involve balance and gentle resistance to support bone strength.

- Combine mindful breathing with physical exercise by pacing your breath with each movement, enhancing both mental calm and physical resilience.

Consistent mindfulness practices contribute significantly to better stress management and improved overall health outcomes. Regular engagement in mindfulness can lead to lower levels of anxiety and depression, conditions often associated with chronic diseases like osteoporosis. Lower stress levels directly translate to less frequent and intense flare-ups of cortisol, protecting bone integrity.

Therefore, embedding mindfulness in every aspect of your day-to-day life isn't just a psychological booster—it's a holistic approach that ensures both mental and physical health. As you adopt these mindfulness practices, you may notice other areas of your life improving too, such as sleep quality and emotional regulation, creating a positive feedback loop that supports your overall wellness.

Incorporating regular mindfulness practices is easier than one might think and doesn't necessarily require prolonged sessions. Simple practices throughout the day can make a substantial difference. Here's what you can do:

- Start your day with a short mindfulness session. Even five minutes of focused breathing can set a positive tone for the rest of the day.

- Take short breaks during work or daily chores to stretch and breathe mindfully. This will refresh your mind and alleviate built-up tension.

- End your day with a mindfulness reflection. Spend a few minutes recounting things you are grateful for and any positive experiences from your day. This promotes relaxation and a peaceful mindset before bed.

Mindfulness, when integrated thoughtfully into various aspects of daily living, creates a robust framework supporting not just mental health but also physical well-being. Studies have shown that people who are consistently mindful tend to have better immune responses and lower inflammation levels, both critical factors in maintaining strong bones (Chen et al., 2023).

As we explore the relationship between mental well-being and bone health through the lens of mindfulness, it becomes clear that simple, consistent practices can yield profound benefits. By reducing stress, enhancing mental clarity, and embedding mindfulness into our daily routines, we can forge a path toward better bone health and overall well-being.

In all your endeavors to manage osteoporosis, remember that small, consistent actions create significant impact. Embrace mindfulness as a continuous journey, one that nurtures your mind and body, enabling you to live more fully and healthily.

Exploring Breathing Techniques for Bone Regeneration

Breathing well is an underappreciated art, but when practiced correctly, it can offer a multitude of benefits for bone health. Deep breathing exercises are particularly effective in this regard, as they help to oxygenate the body, promoting better circulation and enhancing bone regeneration (Bhonde et al., 2016). Oxygen is crucial not just for maintaining our cells but also for supporting the regrowth and repair of tissues, including bones. When we breathe deeply, our blood becomes more oxygen-rich, which improves its ability to transport essential nutrients to various parts of the body, including the bones.

In terms of practical application, proper breathing techniques can significantly aid in relaxation, reducing tension in the body and indirectly supporting bone health. To achieve relaxation through breathing, here are some steps you might find helpful:

- Start by finding a quiet and comfortable spot where you can sit or lie down without distractions.

- Close your eyes and begin to focus on your breath. Place one hand on your chest and the other on your abdomen. • Inhale deeply through your nose, ensuring that your abdomen rises more than your chest. Hold your breath for a few seconds before exhaling slowly through your mouth. •

Repeat this cycle several times, gradually increasing the duration of your inhales and exhales as you feel more comfortable.

By following these guidelines, you can train your body to relax more efficiently. Relieving tension reduces the production of cortisol, a stress hormone that can negatively impact bone density over time (Woodyard, 2011).

Incorporating breathing exercises into daily routines can also improve lung capacity, vitality, and contribute to overall bone strength. Higher lung capacity ensures that more oxygen reaches your bloodstream, thus serving your bones better. Here's how you can integrate such practices seamlessly into your life:

- Begin your day with a series of deep breathing exercises right after you wake up. This not only sets a positive tone for the day but also helps kickstart your body's oxygen delivery system.

- Include short sessions of focused breathing throughout your day. For instance, taking five minutes at lunchtime to practice can refresh both your mind and body.

- Before going to bed, engage in calming breathing exercises to promote relaxation and prepare your body for restful sleep.

Taking these small steps can have profound impacts on your health, and over time, these habits will become second nature, requiring minimal effort to maintain.

Breathing practices like diaphragmatic breathing or pranayama can be powerful tools for enhancing both mental and physical well-being. Diaphragmatic breathing involves using the diaphragm effectively to draw air deep into the lungs, while pranayama focuses on controlling the breath in ways that influence both the mind and body. To get started:

- Sit or lie down comfortably and place one hand on your chest and the other on your abdomen.

- Breathe in deeply through your nose so that your abdomen pushes outward against your hand while your chest remains relatively still.

- Slowly exhale through pursed lips, allowing your abdomen to fall inward toward your spine.

- Practice this for five to ten minutes each day, gradually aiming to extend the time as you become more comfortable.

Pranayama exercises involve a bit more structure and variety:

- Begin with "Nadi Shodhana" or alternate nostril breathing, which balances the nervous system and enhances mental clarity. Block one nostril while inhaling through the other, and then switch for the exhale, repeating for several cycles.

- Another technique is "Kapalabhati" or skull-shining breath, which consists of rapid, forceful exhales followed by passive inhales. This exercise is energizing and detoxifying but should be approached cautiously by beginners.

Adopting these practices can revolutionize your approach to both mental and physical wellness, providing a natural and accessible way to enhance your quality of life.

The consistent practice of these breathing techniques can support bone regeneration and fortify overall bone health, an assertion supported by emerging research (Memorial Sloan Kettering Cancer Center, 2024). Bones are living tissues that constantly remodel themselves; thus, enhancing their environment can have direct beneficial impacts. This makes incorporating breathing exercises all the more valuable, acting as a straightforward, low-cost intervention to bolster bone vitality.

Deep breathing helps expel toxins from our bodies. During rigorous exercises or yoga, muscles and tissues release metabolic waste products like carbon dioxide, lactic acid, and ammonia. The act of deep breathing facilitates the efficient removal of these wastes, decreasing the burden on our bones and supporting their health indirectly. Proper oxygenation through intensive breathing also ensures that the bone remodeling process remains uninterrupted.

Moreover, as you focus on your breathing, the body enters a state of parasympathetic activation. This state promotes healing, growth, and regeneration. It's like pressing a universal reset button on the physiological stress responses that frequently wear down our systems, particularly the skeletal system (Memorial Sloan Kettering Cancer Center, 2024).

Given the critical interplay between breathing and bone health, it's essential to give mindfulness to our daily respiratory habits. We often breathe shallowly, especially under stress, depriving our bodies of the full spectrum of benefits that come from deep, intentional breathing. Taking control of our breath means taking control of our health, and by extension, our bone health.

Therefore, committing to regular, structured breathing exercises can yield significant dividends over time. Not only does it buoy our mental health, reducing stress and anxiety, but it also plays a crucial role in maintaining and even improving bone density and strength. A synthesis of proper breathing techniques into one's daily routine represents a tangible, proactive step anyone can take towards enhanced health.

Remember, every deep breath you take is more than just an inhale or exhale; it is a powerful, restorative action that contributes actively to your wellbeing. Embrace this simple yet profound practice and experience the multifaceted benefits that go beyond the immediate moment, fostering long-term health and resilience.

Understanding the Impact of Positive Thinking on Bone Strength

Positive thinking and optimism have long been acknowledged for their profound effects on overall health outcomes. Extensive research supports that individuals who maintain a positive outlook tend to experience better physical health, including stronger bone density. This connection is particularly significant when considering the management of osteoporosis.

Our mental state can directly influence our physical well-being through various mechanisms. Studies have shown that positive emotions can reduce the levels of harmful stress hormones like cortisol, which, when elevated over prolonged periods, can lead to decreased bone density (Brunton et al., 2014). By fostering a mindset of positivity and optimism, we can help mitigate some of these detrimental hormonal effects and bolster our body's natural defenses against bone deterioration.

Cultivating a positive mindset is not merely about maintaining sunny thoughts; it is about building resilience and reducing stress, both of which are essential in supporting bone health. Here is how you can cultivate such a mindset effectively:

- Begin by identifying stressors in your life and develop strategies to manage them. This could involve mindfulness practices, such as meditation or yoga, which have been proven to decrease stress levels significantly.

- Regularly engage in activities that bring joy and fulfillment. Spend time with loved ones, pursue hobbies, or engage in creative projects. These activities foster emotional balance and create a sense of purpose.

- When encountering challenges or setbacks, reframe your perspective to see them as opportunities for growth rather than insurmountable obstacles. This shift in thinking can strengthen emotional resilience and reduce the impact of negative stress on your body.

Practicing gratitude can immensely enhance your mental well-being and contribute to better bone strength. Gratitude helps shift focus away from what might be going wrong to what is already good and working in your life. Here's how you can practice gratitude daily:

- Keep a gratitude journal where you write down at least three things you are thankful for each day. This practice can shift your focus towards positive events and experiences, promoting a healthier mental state.

- Take moments throughout the day to verbally express gratitude to others. Whether it's thanking a colleague for their support or telling a family member you appreciate them, these actions reinforce positive connections and foster a supportive environment. • Reflect on challenging experiences and identify any small positives within them. This practice can help you build a resilient mindset, seeing difficulties as opportunities for learning and growth.

Adopting affirmations or visualization techniques is another powerful method to reinforce positive thinking patterns and promote bone health. Affirmations are simple, positive statements that you repeat to yourself to encourage a healthy mindset. Visualization involves mentally picturing positive outcomes to motivate and inspire action. Here's how to incorporate these techniques into your routine:

- Start your day with positive affirmations. For example, "My bones are strong and healthy" or "I am capable of managing my health." Say these out loud or write them down to internalize the message. • Use visualization before engaging in activities that support bone health, like exercising. Picture your bones becoming stronger and more robust with each movement. This mental imagery can boost your motivation and commitment to maintaining physical activity.

- Create a vision board that includes images and words representing your health goals. Place it somewhere visible to remind you daily of your commitment to positive health practices.

The benefits of embracing a positive outlook extend beyond mental well-being; they play a crucial role in managing osteoporosis and maintaining bone strength. Through consistent practice of gratitude, cultivating an optimistic mindset, and using affirmations and visualization techniques, you are taking proactive steps toward better bone health.

It is essential to recognize the interconnected nature of mental and physical health. By prioritizing a positive mindset, you not only enhance your resilience and reduce stress but also support the physiological processes that help maintain strong bones. This holistic approach is vital in the effective management of osteoporosis, ensuring that both mind and body are aligned in the pursuit of better health.

Harnessing the Power of the Mind for Optimal Bone Health

Throughout this chapter, we have delved into the intricate relationship between mental wellbeing and bone health, specifically focusing on strategies to leverage this connection for osteoporosis management. Starting with the impact of chronic stress on bone density, it became clear how elevated cortisol levels can lead to significant bone loss over time. The introduction of mind-body techniques as effective tools to counteract stress-induced bone deterioration has provided actionable pathways for enhancing both mental and physical health.

Revisiting our initial discussion, we explored how activities such as meditation, deep breathing exercises, prayer, and spending time in nature can contribute to lowering cortisol levels, thereby supporting bone health. These practices not only offer relaxation but also promote overall wellness, helping individuals manage stress more effectively and create a favorable environment for bone maintenance and regeneration.

Our current position underscores the profound impact that stress management can have on bone density. By integrating these stress-reducing practices into daily routines, individuals can safeguard their bones against the deleterious effects of chronic stress. However, it's important to recognize that managing stress is an ongoing process. Some readers may be concerned about the practical challenges of maintaining consistent stress management practices amidst busy lives or existing health conditions.

The broader implications of these findings suggest that a holistic approach to osteoporosis management can yield substantial benefits. By addressing both mental and physical health, we create a more comprehensive strategy for combating bone density loss. The consequences extend beyond individual well-being; promoting such integrative approaches can potentially influence public health outcomes, reducing the prevalence and impact of osteoporosis on a larger scale.

As we conclude this chapter, consider the power of small, consistent actions in fostering better health. Embrace the journey of incorporating stress-reducing practices into your life, understanding that each step contributes to stronger bones and enhanced overall wellness. Reflect on how your commitment to mental well-being not only nurtures your body but also enriches your life in myriad ways. The path to optimal health is continuous and multifaceted— every mindful breath, every moment of calm, is a step towards a healthier, more resilient you.

References

Global Health NOW. (2017). *The Role for Mindfulness in Public Health*. Retrieved from https://globalhealthnow.org/2017-03/role-mindfulness-public-health

Tobias, J. H., Gould, V., Brunton, L., Deere, K., Rittweger, J., & Lipperts, M. (2014). *Physical Activity and Bone: May the Force be with You. Frontiers in Endocrinology*, 5, Article 20. https://doi.org/10.3389/fendo.2014.00020

Woodyard, C. (2011). *Exploring the therapeutic effects of yoga and its ability to increase quality of life. International Journal of Yoga*, 4(2), 49. https://doi.org/10.4103/0973-6131.85485

Li, H., Jiang, H., Wang, J., Zhou, J., Liang, H., Chen, G., Guo, Z., Yang, S., & Zhang, Y. (2023).
*Effects of Mind-Body Exercises for Osteoporosis in Older Adults: A Systematic Review and
Meta-analysis of Randomized Controlled Trials. Geriatric Orthopaedic Surgery &
Rehabilitation*, 14(10). https://doi.org/10.1177/21514593231195237

<div class="hanging-indent">Memorial Sloan Kettering Cancer Center. (2024). <i>Breathing Exercises</i>. <i>Retrieved from</i> <a href="https://www.mskcc.org/cancer-care/patienteducation/breathing-exercises">https://www.mskcc.org/cancer-care/patient-education/breathingexercises</a></div>

Ng, J.-S., & Chin, K.-Y. (2021). *Potential mechanisms linking psychological stress to bone health. International Journal of Medical Sciences*, 18(3), 604. https://doi.org/10.7150/ijms.50680

Kelly, R. R., McDonald, L. T., Jensen, N. R., Sidles, S. J., & LaRue, A. C. (2019). *Impacts of psychological stress on osteoporosis:*

Clinical implications and treatment interactions. Frontiers in Psychiatry, 10, 200. https://doi.org/10.3389/fpsyt.2019.00200

Bone Health & Osteoporosis Foundation. (2015). *Overall Health. Bone Health & Osteoporosis Foundation*. Retrieved from https://www.bonehealthandosteoporosis.org/patients/treatment/overall-health/

<div class="hanging-indent">Zhang, Y., Wang, Z., Lu, M., Wang, Q., & Wang, H. (2020). <i>Effects of mind-body exercises for osteoporosis in older adults: Protocol for systematic review and Bayesian network meta-analysis of randomized controlled trials</i>. <i>Medicine</i>, 99(11). <a href="https://doi.org/10.1097/MD.0000000000019426">https://doi.org/10.1097/MD.000000000 0019426</a></div>

Shree, N., & Bhonde, R. R. (2016). *Can yoga therapy stimulate stem cell trafficking from bone marrow?. Journal of Ayurveda and Integrative Medicine*, 7(3), 181. https://doi.org/10.1016/j.jaim.2016.07.003

Chapter 9

Preventative Strategies for Osteoporosis

Maintaining strong bones throughout life is a goal many of us share, yet it's often not until we face issues like fractures or a diagnosis of osteoporosis that we prioritize bone health. The clarity of hindsight reminds us that preventive measures could have made all the difference. Imagine feeling confident in your bone health, knowing you took steps early on to ensure strength and resilience. This sense of security isn't reserved for a select few; it's attainable for everyone with the right knowledge and habits.

Osteoporosis silently erodes bone density over time, transforming what were once robust structures into fragile frameworks susceptible to breaks and fractures. A single fall or minor accident can lead to significant disability, altering one's quality of life in profound ways. Consider the common scenario of a person who has always been active, only to find themselves sidelined by a hip fracture. This unfortunate reality isn't just about physical pain; it imposes emotional and social challenges as well. Lives are disrupted, independence is compromised, and the path to recovery can be long and arduous. Early intervention, such as weight-bearing exercises during childhood and consistent nutritional support, can dramatically reduce these risks.

In this chapter, we will explore practical strategies that can help prevent osteoporosis and maintain optimal bone health throughout life. You'll learn how activities like walking, running, and playing sports can fortify your bones from a young age. We'll delve into dietary recommendations, emphasizing the importance of calcium and vitamin D, and provide guidelines for incorporating these nutrients into daily meals. Additionally, the role of regular physical activity at different life stages will be highlighted, offering actionable steps for adults striving to maintain or improve their bone strength. By adopting these proactive measures, you'll be better equipped to safeguard your bone health and enjoy a more active, fulfilling life.

Early Interventions for Bone Health

Engaging in weight-bearing exercises from a young age can help build strong bones and reduce the risk of osteoporosis in later years. Many people think of skeletal health as something to consider only when we're older, but it's actually much more effective to start early. When you engage in activities like walking, running, or playing sports such as soccer and basketball during your childhood and teen years, you're essentially laying down a solid foundation for your bones. These activities put stress on the bones in a healthy way, prompting them to get stronger and denser.

Guidelines for incorporating weight-bearing exercises:

- Encourage children to participate in daily physical activities that involve running, jumping, and other movements that support bone strength.

- Make exercise fun by integrating games and sports into their routine rather than making it feel like a chore.

- Schools and community programs should provide opportunities for kids to stay active through organized sports and physical education classes.

- Parents can lead by example, participating in physical activities with their children to reinforce the importance of regular exercise.

Ensuring adequate intake of calcium and vitamin D during childhood and adolescence is crucial for optimal bone development and future bone health. Calcium acts like the building blocks of bones while Vitamin D is the mason that helps put these blocks together. For children aged 9 to 18, a dietary intake of 1,300 mg of calcium per day and at least 600 IU of Vitamin D is recommended (Osteoporosis Prevention Starts Early - OrthoInfo - AAOS, n.d.). Achieving these levels isn't always straightforward, especially given modern dietary habits.

Guidelines for ensuring adequate calcium and vitamin D intake:

- Include calcium-rich foods like dairy products, leafy green vegetables, and fortified foods in daily diets from an early age.

- Ensure that children spend time outdoors engaging in physical activities, helping them naturally synthesize Vitamin D from sunlight exposure.

- If needed, consult with a healthcare provider about appropriate dietary supplements to fill any gaps in nutrition.

- Educate teenagers on the importance of not skipping meals and incorporating nutritious foods into their daily lives.

Educating parents and caregivers on the significance of incorporating bone-healthy foods like dairy products, leafy greens, and fortified foods in children's diets is imperative. Dietary habits formed in childhood often carry over into adulthood. By focusing on bone-healthy foods, parents can ensure that their children are well-equipped to fight off bone diseases in the future. Foods rich in calcium include dairy products like milk, cheese, and yogurt, while leafy greens like spinach and kale also offer good sources. Additionally, many cereals and orange juices are fortified with both calcium and Vitamin D, making them convenient options.

Emphasizing the role of regular physical activity in maintaining bone strength throughout different life stages remains essential. The reality of life is that peak bone mass is typically achieved by the age of 30. From then on, our bones gradually lose density if we don't take proactive measures to maintain them. This doesn't mean it's too late for those who haven't been active earlier; there's ample evidence to suggest that even older adults can improve their bone health with consistent activity.

For adults, including weight-bearing exercises and resistance training in their routines can be incredibly beneficial. Activities such as hiking, dancing, and lifting weights not only keep the bones strong but also contribute to overall well-being. It's never too late to start, and small steps can make significant differences.

Guidelines for maintaining bone strength through regular physical activity:

- Incorporate activities like brisk walking, jogging, or hiking into daily routines.

- Engage in resistance training exercises such as light weightlifting or body-weight exercises several times a week.

- Participate in group fitness classes or community sports leagues to stay motivated and social.

- Stretch regularly to maintain flexibility and balance, which can prevent falls and related fractures.

The key takeaway is clear: early interventions and lifestyle habits play a significant role in preventing osteoporosis and promoting long-term bone health. Personal responsibility is fundamental, yet societal structures—like schools, employers, and healthcare providers—also have roles to play. On a micro level, individual choices about diet, physical activity, and lifestyle significantly impact one's bone health trajectory. While on a macro level, policies that encourage safe, accessible outdoor spaces for exercise and public health campaigns promoting nutritional education can make a real difference.

In sum, each of us holds the potential to shape our bone health outcomes through mindful, evidence-driven choices. The blend of personal initiative coupled with community and policy support establishes a robust foundation for lifelong wellness. Every step taken today, whether it's opting for a healthier meal or choosing to take the stairs, inches us closer to a more resilient tomorrow—one where strong bones fortify both our bodies and our spirits.

By prioritizing bone health early and consistently throughout our lives, we create a lasting legacy of strength and vitality. So lace up those sneakers, reach for that balanced plate, and look forward to a future where your bones carry you confidently through every adventure life throws your way.

Importance of Regular Bone Density Tests

Bone density tests, especially through dual-energy X-ray absorptiometry (DXA) scans, are critical tools in assessing bone health and identifying the potential risks of osteoporosis before it leads to significant bone loss. These tests work by using low-level X-rays to measure the amount of calcium and other bone minerals packed into a segment of bone, usually focusing on areas prone to fractures such as the spine, hip, and forearm. This method helps pinpoint even small decreases in bone density, providing an early warning system that can be instrumental in taking preemptive actions against osteoporosis.

Now, when should you consider getting these bone density tests? The frequency and age at which you start testing depend largely on individual risk factors and your health history. Here's what you can do to figure out when and how often you should be tested for optimal bone health: •   First, talk to your doctor about any risk factors you may have. Risk factors include family history of osteoporosis, previous fractures, long-term use of medications like steroids, and conditions like rheumatoid arthritis or thyroid diseases.

- Second, based on your specific situation, your doctor might recommend starting bone density tests as early as age 50 if you have significant risk factors or around age 65 for women and 70 for men with no additional risk factors.

- Third, repeat tests should align with the severity of your baseline test results and ongoing risk assessment. Those with moderate osteopenia might need a follow-up every 5 years, while individuals with severe osteopenia or initial signs of osteoporosis could benefit from annual testing.

- Fourth, incorporate lifestyle changes and therapies advised by your healthcare provider to improve bone health between tests.

Understanding the significance of early detection through bone density tests is another critical point. Catching osteoporosis in its nascent stages allows for timely interventions that can significantly delay or prevent the progression of the disease. For instance, dietary changes to increase calcium and vitamin D intake, the introduction of weight-bearing exercises, and potentially the use of medications can all be more effective when started early.

When you receive your bone density test results, it's important to understand what they mean for your future bone health. The results are typically presented as T-scores and Z-scores. A T-score compares your bone density to that of a healthy young adult of your gender. Here's a simple breakdown:

- A T-score of -1 and above is considered normal.

- A T-score between -1 and -2.5 indicates osteopenia, a condition of lower than normal bone density that precedes osteoporosis.

- A T-score of -2.5 and below is generally indicative of osteoporosis.

Meanwhile, the Z-score compares your bone density to others in your age group, sex, and size. If your Z-score is significantly lower than average, further medical evaluation might be required to pinpoint any underlying causes.

These scores play a crucial role in shaping the preventive measures and treatment plans you'll adopt moving forward. For example, someone diagnosed with osteopenia might focus on lifestyle interventions, such as diet and exercise, whereas someone with osteoporosis might require more aggressive treatments, including prescription medications like bisphosphonates or hormone-related therapies.

To sum up, regular bone density testing is not just a diagnostic tool but a proactive approach to maintaining optimal bone health. By understanding when to begin testing based on your unique risks, interpreting the results correctly, and acting on early detections, you can significantly mitigate the adverse effects of osteoporosis. Remember, prevention is always better than cure, especially with a condition as silent yet impactful as osteoporosis.

If your doctor suspects you have osteoporosis, a bone density test can assess your bone strength. Learn about the risks and results of this procedure (Mayo Clinic, 2022).

By integrating these guidelines into your routine, you're taking essential steps towards preserving your bone health and overall well-being. This comprehensive approach not only aims to enhance your quality of life but also ensures that you remain active and independent for as long as possible.

Fall Prevention Techniques for Seniors

Maintaining a safe home environment is crucial for seniors to minimize the risk of falls and fractures. It's important to be proactive in identifying potential hazards around the house and taking steps to eliminate them. Removing clutter, such as loose rugs and electrical cords from walkways, can significantly reduce tripping risks. Additionally, installing grab bars in the bathroom and handrails on both sides of staircases provides extra support where it's needed most (National Institute on Aging, n.d.). Night lights in hallways and bedrooms ensure visibility during nighttime trips, preventing accidents due to poor lighting.

Here is what you can do in order to achieve this goal:

- Look around your home for items that could pose a tripping hazard, like clutter or loose rugs, and remove or secure them.

- Install supportive aids such as grab bars in the bathroom and along stairways to provide additional stability.

- Use night lights in hallways, bathrooms, and bedrooms to improve visibility during the night.

- Ensure that floors are always dry and clean up spills immediately to prevent slipping.

Balance and strength exercises play a vital role in improving stability and reducing the likelihood of falls among older adults. Regular physical activity, as simple as walking or participating in a gentle exercise program like tai chi, can enhance muscle strength and coordination. Balance exercises, specifically, target the body's ability to maintain steadiness, which is critical in fall prevention. For instance, standing on one foot while holding onto a sturdy surface can gradually improve balance. A consistent routine combining these exercises ensures that seniors stay active and their bodies remain strong, thus lowering the chances of falling.

Here's how you can incorporate these exercises effectively:

- Start with basic balance exercises like standing on one foot while holding a sturdy chair or countertop for support.

- Engage in low-impact activities such as walking, water workouts, or tai chi, which are excellent for overall strength and flexibility.

- If you're new to exercising, consider consulting a physical therapist who can tailor an exercise program specific to your needs and abilities.

- Gradually increase the intensity and duration of your workouts as your strength and balance improve.

Proper footwear, lighting, and home modifications are essential components in minimizing the risk of tripping or slipping accidents. Ensuring that shoes have non-slip soles and fit well can prevent many fall incidents. Avoid high heels, floppy slippers, or shoes with slick bottoms. Instead, opt for sturdy, supportive footwear that provides good grip. Improving home lighting also plays a significant part; brightening dark areas and ensuring light switches are easily accessible can prevent missteps.

For home modifications:

- Choose flat shoes with nonskid soles over high heels, slippers, or sandals with smooth bottoms.

- Update lighting in your living spaces by adding brighter bulbs, especially in areas prone to shadows.

- Place lamps within reach of your bed and install glow-in-the-dark or illuminated switches to make navigating at night easier.

- Make use of assistive devices, such as canes or walkers if recommended by your healthcare provider, to help maintain balance and mobility.

Incorporating fall prevention strategies into daily routines and lifestyle habits is another key element to enhancing overall safety and mobility. Developing a habit of regular exercise, maintaining a clutter-free home, and using assistive devices can all be woven seamlessly into everyday life. Activities such as yoga or Pilates not only contribute to physical health but also instill a sense of discipline and mindfulness, which can be beneficial in preventing falls.

Here are simple changes you can adopt:

- Integrate balance and strength exercises into your daily schedule, even if it's just a few minutes each day.

  Regularly check and maintain your home environment to ensure it remains free of hazards.

  Use backpacks or shoulder bags to keep your hands free, allowing you to hold onto railings or other supports.

- Be mindful of any side effects from medications that might affect your balance, and discuss any concerns with your healthcare provider.

- Stay hydrated and eat a balanced diet to keep your energy levels up, as weakness and fatigue can lead to falls.

The importance of fall prevention measures cannot be overstated when it comes to protecting seniors against fractures and enabling them to maintain their independence as they age. Statistics indicate that more than one in four people aged 65 or older fall each year, yet many of these falls can be prevented with thoughtful, proactive measures (National Institute on Aging, n.d.). By educating seniors about creating a safe home environment, emphasizing the significance of balance and strength exercises, choosing appropriate footwear, and integrating preventative strategies into daily routines, we collectively work toward a safer and healthier future for our aging population.

This approach is not just about avoiding injuries but also about empowering seniors to live their lives fully, confidently, and independently. Both empirical evidence and practical wisdom align in showing us that these seemingly small steps can lead to substantial improvements in quality of life. It's a cooperative effort

-

-

-

involving families, healthcare providers, and communities to ensure that everyone has the resources and knowledge to stay safe and thrive.

Ultimately, it's about striking a balance between promoting individual freedom and ensuring social responsibility. Through informed decision-making and consistent application of these preventative measures, seniors can enjoy a higher degree of autonomy without compromising on safety. This equilibrium is crucial, as it acknowledges the complexity of aging while embracing the capabilities and dignity of older adults.

Creating a Bone-Friendly Home Environment

Creating a bone-friendly home environment is crucial for promoting optimal bone health and reducing the risk of injuries, especially as we age. In today's world, where osteoporosis and other bone density problems are increasingly common, taking proactive measures at home can be lifechanging.

Designing living spaces with good lighting, minimal clutter, and non-slip surfaces is essential to promote safety and prevent falls at home. Falls are a significant cause of fractures among individuals with osteoporosis. To create a safer environment:

> Ensure your home is well-lit. This makes it easier to see obstacles that could cause tripping. Nightlights in hallways and bathrooms can be particularly helpful.

-

-

-

    Keep spaces free of clutter. This means regularly picking up items like shoes, magazines, or toys that might accumulate on the floor.

    Install non-slip mats in areas prone to getting wet, such as bathrooms and kitchens. Additionally, consider using non-slip pads under rugs to prevent them from slipping and causing falls.

Encouraging the use of supportive furniture, handrails, and grab bars in high-risk areas like bathrooms and staircases can prevent accidents. These additions can help maintain balance and provide support when needed most. Here's what you can do:

- Choose chairs and sofas with firm cushions and armrests to make it easier to sit down and stand up.

- Install handrails along both sides of staircases. They should be sturdy and easy to grip.

- Place grab bars in the bathroom, especially near the toilet and inside the shower or bathtub. Make sure they are installed correctly and can support weight.

- Opt for a stable shower chair and a handheld shower head to reduce the need to stand for extended periods while showering.

Implementing ergonomic practices and proper lifting techniques reduces strain on bones and joints during daily activities. Many of us underestimate the impact of poor ergonomics and incorrect lifting on our musculoskeletal health. Taking these steps can help:

-

-

-

- When lifting objects, use your legs rather than your back. Bend at the knees and keep your back straight.

- Avoid twisting your body while carrying heavy loads. Turn your whole body instead.

- Use tools and equipment designed to minimize strain, such as long-handled reachers for picking things up off the floor or high shelves.

- Adjust the height of your workspaces to avoid stooping or overreaching. For example, ensure kitchen countertops are at a comfortable height for food preparation.

Emphasizing the importance of ergonomics, posture, and body mechanics in maintaining bone health and preventing musculoskeletal issues cannot be overstated. Good posture supports bone alignment and reduces unnecessary stress on bones and muscles. Everyday habits have a substantial effect:

Maintain an upright posture when sitting and standing. Your ears should align with your shoulders, which should align with your hips.

Sit with your feet flat on the ground and your knees at a right angle. If necessary, use a footrest.

Take regular breaks to stretch and move around if you're sitting for long periods.

- Invest in ergonomic office chairs and desks if you spend a lot of time working at a computer. These can help support the natural curve of your spine and reduce strain.

-

-

-

All these adjustments contribute significantly to creating a bone-friendly home environment that supports overall safety, well-being, and bone health for individuals of all ages. It's not just about making changes for those already suffering from bone density issues; it's about fostering a proactive approach to prevent such conditions from developing in the first place.

Regular physical activity is another cornerstone of maintaining bone health. Activities that emphasize balance and strength training can help build and maintain bone mass, reducing the risk of falls and fractures. According to evidence (Physical Activity for Best Bone Health, n.d.), people who engage in weight-bearing exercises like walking, running, or dancing have stronger musculoskeletal systems, which lower their risk of osteoporosis-related falls.

Incorporating physical activity into your lifestyle does more than just strengthen bones. It enhances neuromuscular coordination, which plays a critical role in fall prevention. Activities that require your muscles to work against gravity, such as stair climbing, hiking, or even gardening, are highly beneficial. While swimming and biking are excellent for cardiovascular health, they do not offer the same bone-strengthening benefits.

Furthermore, diet plays an essential role in bone health. Adequate calcium and vitamin D intake are vital for maintaining bone density. However, other nutrients also play a part. Potassium-rich fruits and vegetables help in reducing calcium loss through urine, supporting overall bone strength (Deng et al., 2004). Hence, a well-balanced diet rich in these nutrients is advisable.

Building healthy habits early can lead to significant long-term benefits. Adolescents, for instance, should focus on achieving peak bone mass, which typically occurs by late adolescence. Failure to do

-

-

-

so can leave one with less bone reserve to withstand the normal losses that occur later in life ((US), 2004). Thus, ensuring children and teenagers consume sufficient calcium and participate in physical activities like sports or dance can lay a strong foundation for lifelong bone health.

To sum up, creating a bone-friendly home environment involves thoughtful design and proactive measures. Good lighting, minimal clutter, non-slip surfaces, supportive furniture, and ergonomic practices all serve to reduce injury risks. Emphasizing regular physical activity and a nutrientrich diet further bolsters bone health. Combining these elements creates a safe and supportive environment conducive to maintaining strong and healthy bones throughout life.

Summarizing Preventative Approaches for Lifelong Bone Health

In this chapter, we explored various proactive measures that can significantly impact bone health throughout life. Starting from a young age, engaging in weight-bearing exercises such as walking, running, or playing sports is crucial in building strong bones and reducing the risk of osteoporosis. We've discussed strategies to make physical activities enjoyable for children and highlighted the importance of schools and community programs in supporting an active lifestyle.

We also emphasized the necessity of proper nutrition, particularly calcium and Vitamin D, crucial building blocks for developing healthy bones. Ensuring a balanced diet that includes these nutrients through food or supplements can lay a solid foundation for lifelong bone health. Parents play an essential role in instilling these dietary habits early on, setting the stage for a future without bone-related ailments.

As individuals age, maintaining bone density becomes increasingly vital. Regular physical activity, including resistance training and balance exercises, helps preserve bone mass and prevent falls. Older adults can continue to benefit from starting or maintaining an active routine tailored to their capabilities, ensuring ongoing bone strength and overall well-being.

Additionally, regular bone density tests are valuable tools for early detection and management of potential osteoporosis. These tests can guide timely interventions, significantly mitigating the severity of bone loss. Understanding the results and working with healthcare providers to adopt necessary lifestyle changes or treatments can prevent further deterioration of bone health.

Creating a safe home environment also emerged as a critical factor, especially for seniors. By removing tripping hazards, installing supportive aids like grab bars, and choosing proper footwear, we can greatly reduce the likelihood of falls and fractures. Ergonomic practices and mindful body mechanics further support bone and joint health during daily activities.

While individual choices in diet, exercise, and lifestyle are fundamental, societal structures also have roles to play in promoting bone health. Schools, employers, and healthcare providers can all contribute by creating environments that support active, healthy lifestyles. Public health campaigns and policies that encourage accessible outdoor spaces for exercise and offer nutritional education can further bolster these efforts.

Ultimately, the path to optimal bone health is a blend of personal responsibility and community support. Each small choice—whether it's participating in physical activities, maintaining a nutritious diet, or making home modifications—builds towards a stronger, healthier future. Fostering these habits early and sustaining them throughout life ensures not just physical resilience but also the confidence to live fully and independently.

By committedly prioritizing bone health, we can look forward to a lifetime where our bones support us through every adventure, challenge, and joy. The steps we take now, both individually and collectively, pave the way for a more robust tomorrow. So let's take each step mindfully, nurturing our bones, and embracing a future filled with vitality and strength.

References

Mayo Clinic. (2022). *Fall prevention: Simple tips to prevent falls. Mayo Clinic*. Retrieved from https://www.mayoclinic.org/healthy-lifestyle/healthy-aging/in-depth/fall-prevention/art20047358

OrthoInfo - AAOS. (n.d.). *Osteoporosis Prevention Starts Early*. Retrieved from https://www.orthoinfo.aaos.org/en/staying-healthy/osteoporosis-prevention-starts-early/

Pennsylvania State University. (n.d.). *Physical Activity for Best Bone Health.* Retrieved from https://extension.psu.edu/physical-activity-for-best-bone-health

Mayo Clinic. (2022). *Bone density test.* Retrieved from https://www.mayoclinic.org/testsprocedures/bone-density-test/about/pac-20385273

Office of the Surgeon General (US). (2004). *Determinants of Bone Health. Bone Health and Osteoporosis - NCBI Bookshelf.* Retrieved from https://www.ncbi.nlm.nih.gov/books/NBK45503/

Kling, J. M., Clarke, B. L., & Sandhu, N. P. (2014). *Osteoporosis prevention, screening, and treatment: A review. Journal of Women's Health*, 23(7), 563. https://doi.org/10.1089/jwh.2013.4611

Office of the Surgeon General (US). (2004). *Population-based Approaches to Promote Bone Health. Bone Health and Osteoporosis - NCBI Bookshelf.* Retrieved from https://www.ncbi.nlm.nih.gov/books/NBK45512/

National Institute on Aging. (n.d.). *Six Tips To Help Prevent Falls.* Retrieved from https://www.nia.nih.gov/health/falls-and-falls-prevention/six-tips-help-prevent-falls

National Institute on Aging. (n.d.). *Falls and Fractures in Older Adults: Causes and Prevention.* Retrieved from https://www.nia.nih.gov/health/falls-and-falls-prevention/falls-and-fracturesolder-adults-causes-and-prevention

Office of the Surgeon General (US). (2004). *A Public Health Approach to Promote Bone Health. Bone Health and Osteoporosis.* Retrieved from https://www.ncbi.nlm.nih.gov/books/NBK45518/

Chapter 10

Empowering Self-Care Practices

Self-care, often dismissed as a modern luxury, forms the cornerstone of maintaining robust bone health. Picture this: a life free from the nagging worry about fractures or the relentless ache of osteoporosis. Empowering yourself with simple, daily practices can transform that picture into reality. Imagine the confidence that comes with knowing you're actively nurturing your bones, ensuring they stay strong and resilient for years to come. This chapter invites you to take charge of your well-being through actionable, personalized strategies.

Bone health is not merely about avoiding breaks and fractures; it's about fostering resilience from within. Many adults today face the challenge of reduced bone density, which, if left unchecked, can lead to conditions like osteoporosis. For example, older adults might find themselves increasingly cautious about activities they once enjoyed due to fear of injury. Simple tasks like walking up stairs or bending to pick up a grandchild become fraught with risk. This decline in bone strength isn't inevitable, though. With the right self-care practices, including exercise and nutrition adjustments, you can fortify your bones against deterioration.

In this chapter, we will explore various self-care techniques designed to bolster bone health. From developing a personalized plan that fits seamlessly into your lifestyle to incorporating effective exercises and dietary choices, we'll provide you with practical steps to enhance your bone strength. You'll learn how specific activities and nutrition can make a significant difference, and discover the role of regular self-assessment tools in tracking your progress. Additionally, we'll underline the importance of professional guidance to tailor your approach further. By the end, you'll be well-equipped to integrate these practices into your daily routine, thus empowering yourself to achieve optimal bone health naturally.

Developing a Personalized Bone Health Plan

Taking charge of your bone health starts with understanding what your personal goals should be and how to tailor them to fit your unique needs and lifestyle. It's not just about following a generic plan; it's about developing a strategy that's customized for you. The first step is to identify what you aim to achieve with your bone health. Are you looking to maintain current bone density, prevent future bone deterioration, or perhaps even improve bone strength? Knowing your objective will guide what steps you incorporate into your daily routine.

If you are old enough ,you can take advantage of Silver Sneakers which is available at most Gyms.

A significant part of achieving these personalized goals is integrating specific exercises known to strengthen bones. Weight-bearing exercises like walking, jogging, and even climbing stairs play a crucial role in maintaining bone density. Walking, for example, is particularly recommended to help prevent conditions such as osteoporosis (Director, 2019). Additionally, resistance training using free weights or exercise machines can enhance bone strength by making muscles pull on the bones during workouts.

Alongside physical activity, nutrition is a cornerstone of any effective bone health plan. Your body relies heavily on calcium and vitamin D to build and maintain strong bones. For adults aged 19 to 50 and men up to age 70, the Recommended Dietary Allowance (RDA) for calcium is 1,000 milligrams (mg) per day. For women over 51 and men over 71, this increases to 1,200 mg daily (Mayo Clinic, 2022). Sources of calcium include dairy products, broccoli, kale, sardines, and fortified foods like soy milk. Vitamin D helps your body absorb calcium and can be obtained from diet sources such as oily fish, mushrooms, eggs, and fortified cereals, as well as from sunlight exposure.

Here is what you can do to ensure you're getting enough of these vital nutrients:

- Incorporate a variety of calcium-rich foods into each meal. Think beyond milk – include leafy greens, nuts, and seeds. • Ensure you're getting enough vitamin D through both diet and responsible sun exposure. Consult your doctor if supplements might be needed.

- Plan meals that are balanced and nutrient-dense, focusing on whole foods over processed ones.

Consistency is key when adopting new habits for bone health. Establishing a daily routine that includes both appropriate exercises and nutrient intake sets a foundation for long-term success. Begin with small, manageable changes—perhaps starting with a 20-minute walk daily and gradually adding weight training twice a week. Over time, these activities will become a seamless part of your everyday life.

Self-assessment tools are another useful way to track progress and make necessary adjustments.
Interactive online tools, such as those available from the National Institutes of Health
Osteoporosis and Related Bone Diseases~National Resource Center, provide valuable feedback tailored to your responses (Director, 2019). These tools help you understand factors that may increase your risk for conditions like osteoporosis and ways to mitigate those

risks. By regularly checking in on your progress, you can see what's working and where you might need to make changes.

Here's how you can effectively use self-assessment tools:

- Use online questionnaires to evaluate your bone health status periodically.

- Track your physical activity and dietary intake in a journal or app to monitor consistency.

- Adjust your exercise and nutrition plans based on the insights gained from these assessments.

In your journey to better bone health, consulting with healthcare professionals is indispensable. Personalized advice from a doctor or a nutritionist can fine-tune your approach and ensure that you're meeting all your dietary and physical needs. A bone density test might be recommended if there's concern about your bone health. This test provides critical information about your bone density levels and helps your doctor decide on any additional measures, such as medication, that might be necessary to slow bone loss (Mayo Clinic, 2022).

Guidance from healthcare professionals can assist you in:

- Understanding the results of a bone density test and what they mean for your health.

- Tailoring an individualized exercise program based on professional recommendations.

- Determining the need for dietary supplements or medications.

When constructing your bone health strategy, remember that personalization, consistency, regular assessment, and professional guidance are the pillars of success. Making these elements a priority elevates the likelihood of achieving and maintaining optimal bone health.

Let's break down these key takeaways:

- Personalization: Tailor your bone health plan to meet your specific goals and lifestyle.

- Consistency: Stick to a regular routine of weight-bearing exercises and nutrient-dense diet.

- Assessment: Regularly utilize self-assessment tools to make informed adjustments.

- Professional Guidance: Seek advice and evaluations from healthcare professionals to ensure you're on the right track.

By focusing on these areas, you'll be well-equipped to take charge of your bone health through effective self-care practices and natural remedies. Remember, the goal is not only to foster economic growth but to prioritize human welfare, ensuring everyone has the capacity to thrive. Your empowered approach to bone health reflects a balance between personal responsibility and the importance of accessing a safety net when needed. Here's to building stronger bones and, with them, a stronger future.

Incorporating Self-Massage Techniques

Incorporating self-massage techniques into your daily routine can be a significant step towards maintaining and improving bone health. This simple yet effective practice not only targets areas prone to bone density loss, such as the spine and hips, but also brings holistic benefits to your overall well-being by enhancing circulation, reducing muscle tension, and promoting relaxation.

Why Self-Massage?

Self-massage is highly advantageous, especially for those dealing with osteoporosis or general bone density issues. It enables you to directly address sore points or areas of discomfort, providing immediate relief and fostering long-term benefits. Massage therapy has been shown to improve joint flexibility and circulation, which are crucial in preventing further bone density deterioration. When applied correctly, self-massage can be particularly beneficial for alleviating pain and stiffness associated with conditions like osteoarthritis (Atkins, 2015).

To get started with self-massage for bone health, focus on areas where bones are most susceptible to density loss. The spine and hips are common concern areas, given their role in maintaining posture and mobility. Targeting these locations through massage can stimulate blood flow and promote nutrient delivery to the bones, thus enhancing their strength and resilience.

Specific Techniques

For an effective self-massage routine aimed at promoting bone health, consider incorporating the following techniques:

- Start with large, vigorous strokes to warm up and prepare your muscles. This step is vital as it helps increase blood flow and loosen up the tissues.

- Use smaller, precise strokes to target specific areas. Apply gentle pressure using your hands, knuckles, or even elbows. For instance, when massaging the spine, use your fingertips to apply circular motions along each side of the spinal column. This technique helps to alleviate tension and foster nutrient-rich blood flow to the vertebrae. • Incorporate deep gliding strokes (effleurage) along the length of your thighs and hips. Place the heel of your hand on your thigh and glide downwards towards the knee while applying moderate pressure. Repeat this motion several times to help soften and lengthen the muscle fibers around your hip joints

(There are many different massage techniques to choose from. Find out which type of massage is best for you., n.d.).

- For areas that are harder to reach, such as the upper back and neck, using massage tools like foam rollers or massage balls can be extremely helpful. Simply roll the tool against the targeted area to break down knots and reduce muscle tightness.

Integrating Self-Massage into Your Routine

Making self-massage part of your daily routine doesn't have to be time-consuming or complicated. In fact, just a few minutes a day can make a significant difference in your bone health and overall well-being. Here are some practical tips for seamlessly incorporating selfmassage into your lifestyle:

- Designate a specific time each day for your self-massage. Mornings and evenings are often the best times because they align well with other self-care activities like stretching or brushing your teeth.

- Use your relaxation time effectively. Consider integrating self-massage into your bedtime routine. This not only ensures you do it regularly but also promotes relaxation, helping you sleep better.

- Pair self-massage with other wellness practices like yoga or meditation. These activities complement each other well, enhancing both physical and mental health. Gentle yoga stretches can further support bone health by improving flexibility and reducing the risk of injuries.

- Keep massage tools readily available. Having items like foam rollers, massage balls, or even a tennis ball within easy reach ensures you are more likely to use them. Place these tools in visible spots around your home or workspace as a constant reminder.

- Listen to your body. Pay attention to how your body responds to the massage. If you feel any pain or discomfort, adjust your pressure or technique accordingly. The goal is to promote healing and relaxation, not to cause additional strain.

Benefits of Self-Massage

The benefits of self-massage extend far beyond immediate physical relief. Here are key advantages you can expect from incorporating self-massage into your routine:

- Improved Circulation: Regular self-massage encourages better circulation, ensuring that your bones receive an adequate supply of nutrients and oxygen necessary for maintaining their density and strength.

- Reduced Muscle Tension: By targeting and relaxing tense muscles, self-massage helps alleviate stress on bones and joints. This can significantly reduce the risk of falls and fractures.

- Enhanced Bone Strength: Stimulating the muscles and tissues surrounding bones can indirectly contribute to bone health by fostering an environment conducive to bone growth and repair.

- Stress Reduction: The act of self-massage itself is incredibly relaxing. Taking a few moments each day to focus on your body can reduce stress levels and improve your overall mood. Lower stress levels have been linked to better bone health as high stress can lead to increased production of cortisol, a hormone that may negatively impact bone density.

Tools and Resources

Various tools can enhance your self-massage experience and make it more effective. Here are some commonly used tools and resources along with tips on how to use them:

- Foam Rollers: Great for larger muscle groups like the thighs and back. Simply place the roller underneath the targeted area and gently roll back and forth, allowing the pressure to relieve muscle tightness and improve circulation.

- Massage Balls: Useful for pinpointing specific areas of tension, especially around the spine or shoulders. Place the ball against the targeted spot and use your body weight to apply pressure, rolling slowly over the area.

- Heat Pads: Applying heat before your massage session can help relax muscles and increase blood flow, making the massage more effective. Use a heating pad or a warm towel for about 10 minutes before starting your self-massage routine.

- Online Tutorials: Numerous online resources provide guided self-massage techniques. Websites, videos, and apps can offer visual aids and step-by-step instructions to ensure you are performing the techniques correctly and safely.

Key Takeaways

Engaging in regular self-massage is a straightforward yet powerful way to support better bone health and overall well-being. Here are the essential points to remember:

- Self-massage improves circulation, which is crucial for transporting nutrients to your bones.

- It helps reduce muscle tension, thereby lowering the stress on your bones and joints.

- Regular self-massage can enhance bone strength indirectly by fostering an optimal environment for bone growth and repair.

- Beyond physical benefits, self-massage promotes relaxation and reduces stress, contributing to better overall health.

Remember, self-massage is not a replacement for professional medical care but a complementary practice that, when done consistently, can significantly improve your quality of life. So why not take charge of your bone health today? Your future self will thank you.

Holistic Strategies for Long-Term Bone Health

Taking proactive steps for your bone health through self-care practices and natural remedies involves adopting various personalized strategies. This chapter has emphasized the importance of integrating specific exercises, a nutrient-rich diet, and using effective self-assessment tools to track progress. Moreover, seeking professional healthcare advice is crucial to tailor your plan further and ensure you're on the right path.

Returning to our opening statement about the need for a customized strategy, it becomes evident that one-size-fits-all plans are insufficient. Each individual's goals and lifestyle factors must be considered to develop an effective bone health regimen. As we have discussed, determining whether you aim to maintain current bone density, prevent deterioration, or improve bone strength is essential to guiding your daily activities.

The consistency of applying weight-bearing exercises, ensuring adequate intake of calcium and vitamin D, and regularly using self-assessment tools cannot be overstated. Establishing these habits as part of your daily routine will set a solid foundation for long-term bone health. Readers should be mindful that while these practices are beneficial, they require ongoing dedication and adjustments based on personal progress and needs.

On a broader scale, the consequences of maintaining good bone health extend beyond individual well-being. Society benefits from reducing the prevalence of osteoporosis and other bone-related issues, which can lessen healthcare costs and improve overall quality of life for many. Furthermore, a community committed to wellness practices fosters an environment where preventive health is prioritized over reactive treatments.

In conclusion, embracing a personalized approach to bone health is a powerful step toward safeguarding your future mobility and quality of life. By consistently incorporating tailored exercises, balanced nutrition, self-assessment, and professional guidance into your routine, you can take charge of your bone health effectively. Remember, bone health is not just a short-term goal but a lifelong commitment. As you adopt and refine these practices, consider how they fit into your broader vision of well-being. Your journey towards stronger bones starts today, and with it, a stronger future awaits.

References

Atkins, D. (2015). *Self-Massage For Knee Pain. Massage Therapy Journal.* Retrieved from https://www.amtamassage.org/publications/massage-therapy-journal/knee-self-massage/

McSwan, J., Gudin, J., Song, X.-J., Plapler, P. G., Betteridge, N. J., Kechemir, H., ... Pickering, G. (2021). *Self-Healing: A Concept for Musculoskeletal Body Pain Management – Scientific Evidence and Mode of Action. Journal of Pain Research,* 14, 2943. https://doi.org/10.2147/JPR.S321037

National Institute of Arthritis and Musculoskeletal and Skin Diseases. (2019). *Take Steps To Improve Your Bone Health. NIAMS.*

Retrieved from https://archive.niams.nih.gov/2010/takesteps-improve-your-bone-health

Arthritis Foundation. (n.d.). *Types of Massage*. Retrieved from https://www.arthritis.org/healthwellness/treatment/complementary-therapies/natural-therapies/types-of-massage

Mayo Clinic. (2022). *How to keep your bones healthy*. Retrieved from https://www.mayoclinic.org/healthy-lifestyle/adult-health/in-depth/bone-health/art-20045060 Office of the Surgeon General (US). (2004). *Population-based Approaches to Promote Bone Health. Bone Health and Osteoporosis*. Retrieved from https://www.ncbi.nlm.nih.gov/books/NBK45512/